The Funny Side Collection
The Fart Side
Windbreaks!
(Expanded Full Blast Edition!)

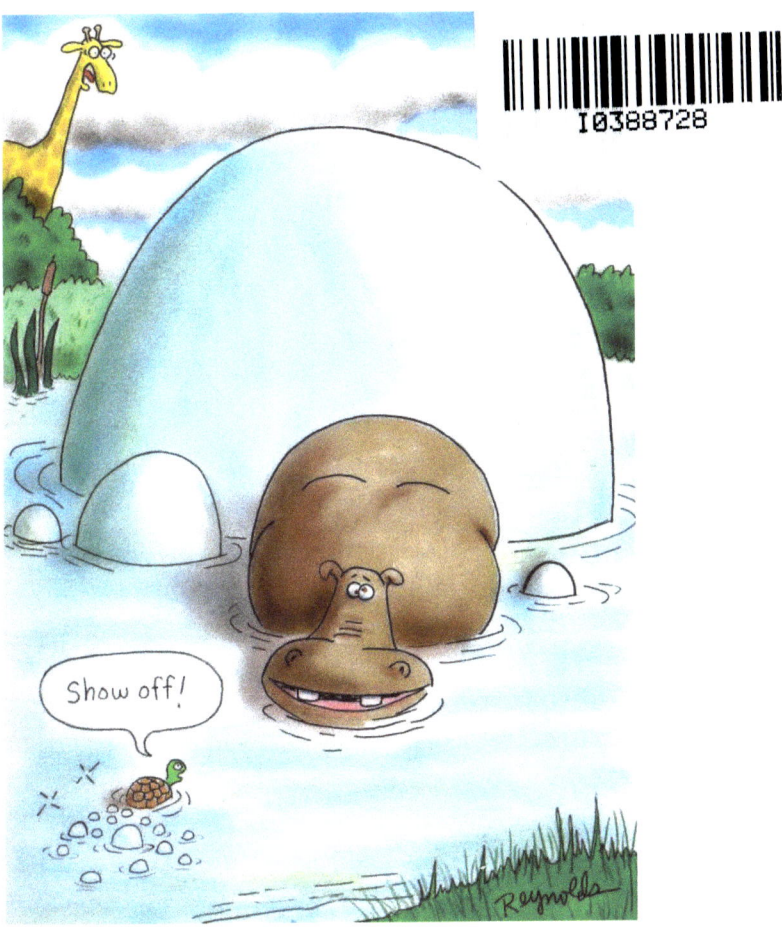

Dan Reynolds
Joseph Weiss, MD

© 2017 Dan Reynolds
       Joseph Weiss, M.D.
       SmartAsk Books
       Rancho Santa Fe, California, USA
       www.smartaskbooks.com

All rights reserved. No part of this book may be reproduced, reused, republished, or retransmitted in any form, or stored in a database or retrieval system, without written permission of the publisher.

ISBN-13: 978-1-943760-59-6 (Color Print Expanded)
ISBN-13: 978-1-943760-60-8 (e-Book Expanded)
ISBN-13: 978-1-943760-54-1 (Color Print Pocket Rocket)
ISBN-13: 978-1-943760-55-8 (e-Book Pocket Rocket)

The Fart Side: Windbreaks!

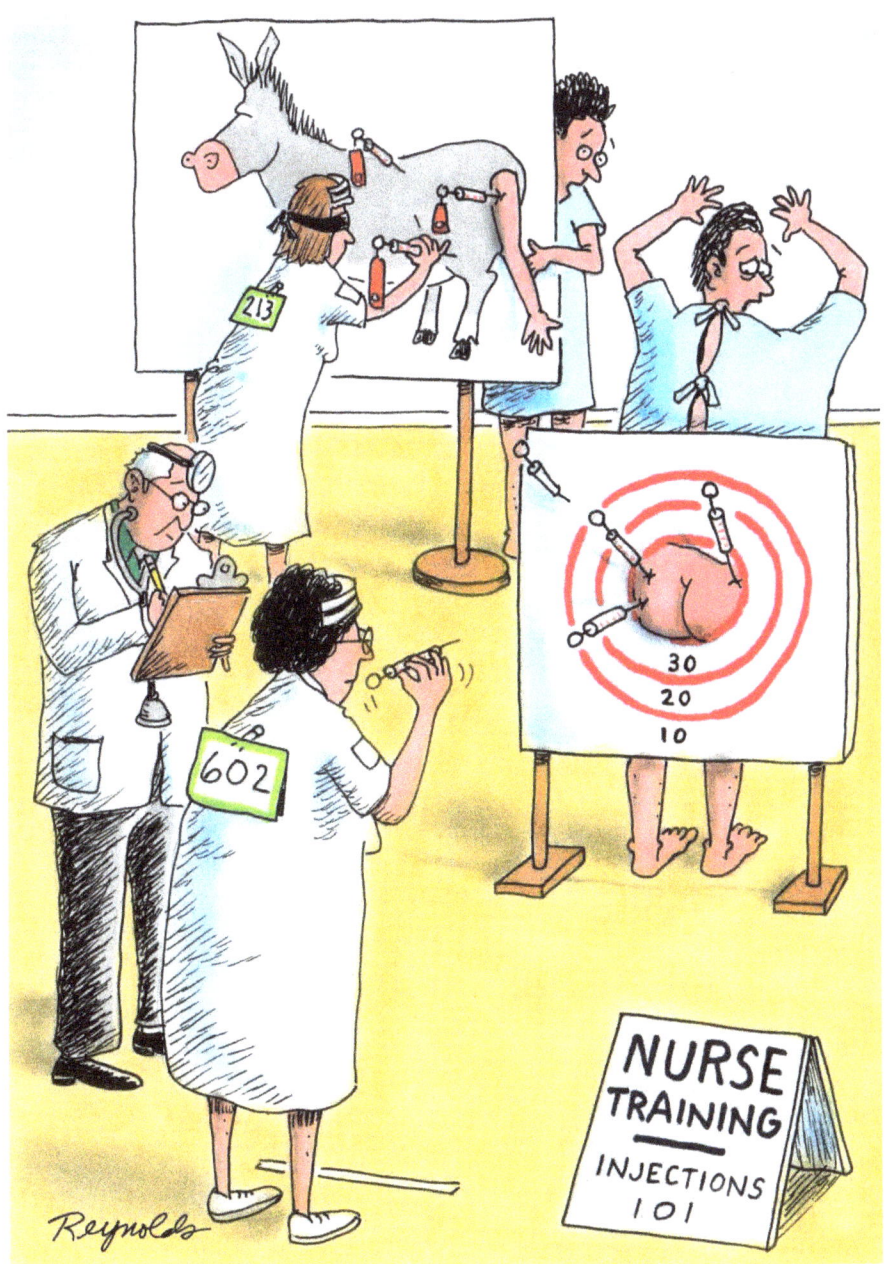

The Funny Side Collection

The fart bubble of a blue whale is so large it can envelope a horse and rider and asphyxiate both.

The small intestine is more than three times as long as the large intestine.

Large quantities of carbon dioxide gas are generated when the stomach contents enter the small intestine.

The farts of carnivores smell more offensive than the farts of vegetarians.

About thirty percent of people produce flammable farts.

It can take your gut flora up to a year to fully repopulate itself after just one course of antibiotics.

Toilet paper must be ten sheets thick to prevent fecal contamination of the hands with wiping.

The Fart Side: Windbreaks!

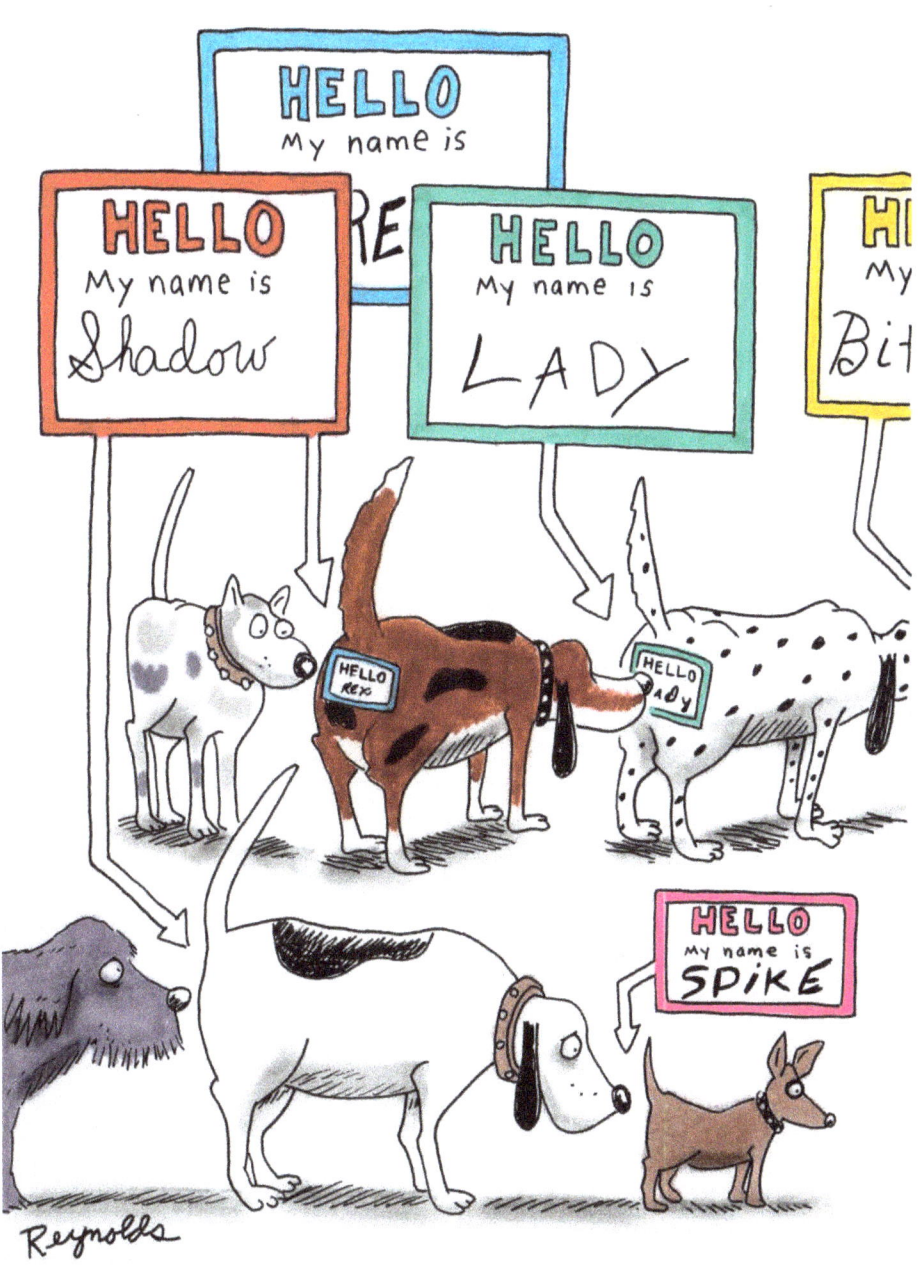

About thirty percent of people enjoy the aroma of their farts.

The largest organ or tissue of the body exposed to the external environment is the gastrointestinal tract.

The total surface area of the gastrointestinal tract exceeds that of a championship tennis court.

The intestines may also commonly be referred to as the alimentary tract, alimentary canal, digestive tract, gastrointestinal (GI) tract, bowels, small bowel, large bowel, hollow viscus, gut, entrails, viscera, or innards.

The liver is the largest organ in the body and performs more than five hundred functions.

Food stays in the stomach for an average of two to three hours.

The Fart Side: Windbreaks!

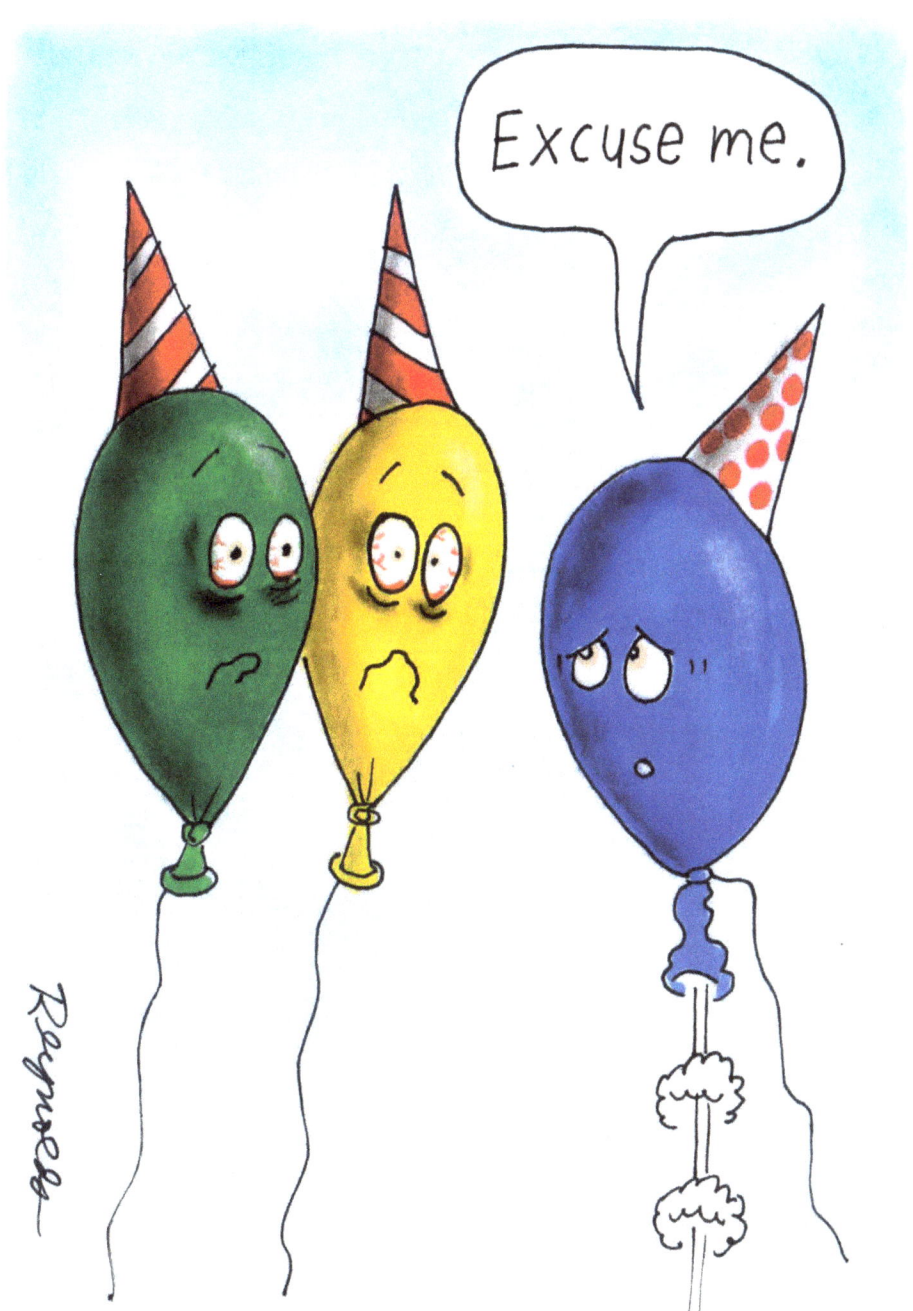

Ninety-five percent of the body's supply of the well-recognized and critically important neurotransmitter serotonin is found in the gut.

The brain and its serotonin receptors contain only five percent of the body's serotonin.

Serotonin receptors are a frequent target of prescription medications such as Prozac (fluoxetine), which are known as a selective serotonin re-uptake inhibitor (SSRI).

The gut and the brain each have fifty percent of the body's supply of dopamine, another important neurotransmitter.

Borborygmus is the name given to audible stomach growls and sounds.

An adult esophagus ranges from 10 to 14 inches in length, and 1 inch in diameter.

The Fart Side: Windbreaks!

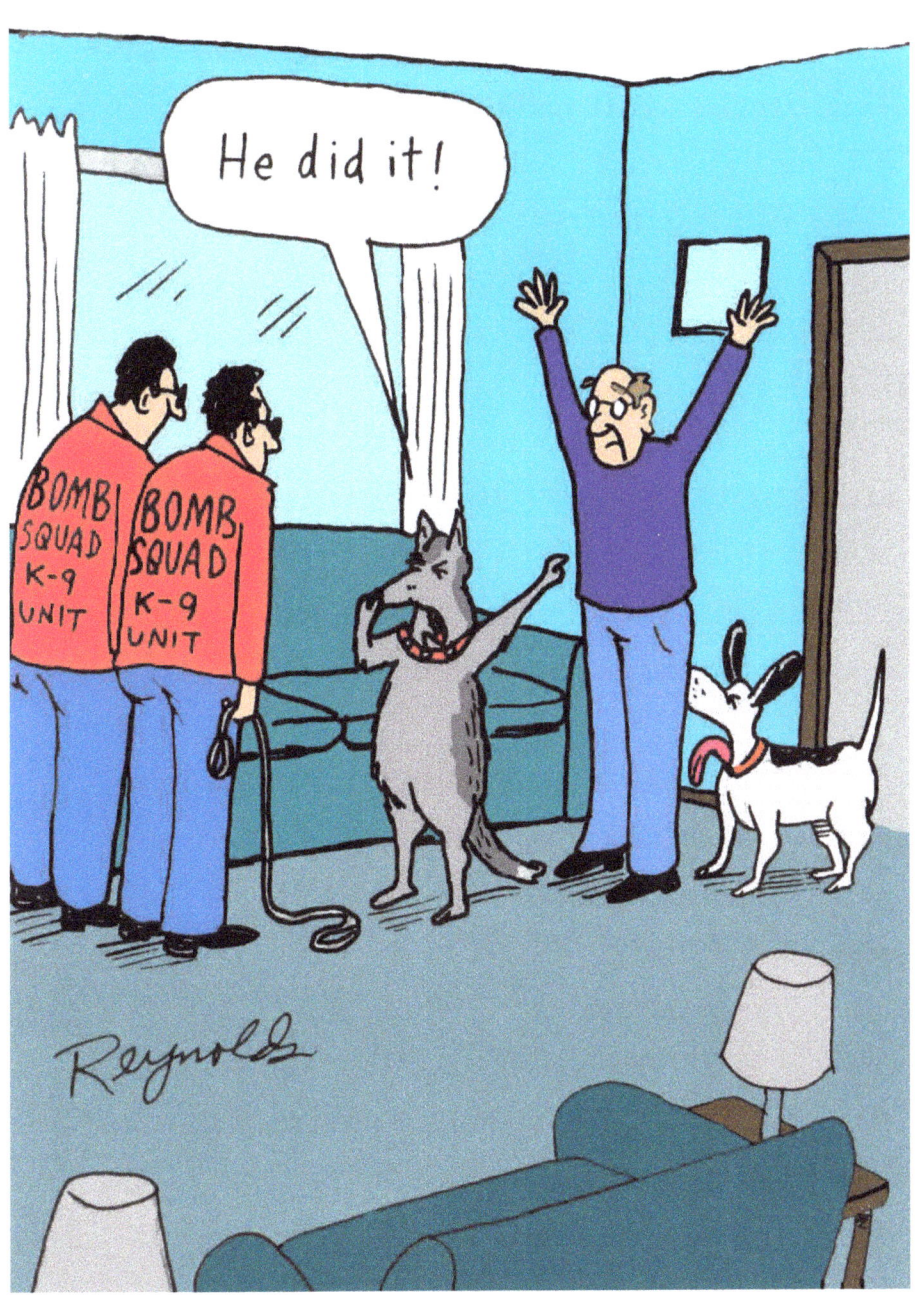

Hydrogen and methane are two gasses produced by the gut microbes that are flammable and explosive.

Hydrogen and methane are odorless.

Hydrogen is lighter than air, and lighter than helium.

The known universe is ninety-nine percent hydrogen and helium, the two lightest elements, and which are nearly always found as gases.

Planets are the extreme astronomical oddity of being comprised of heaver elements of liquids and solids, as well as gasses.

The digestive system is made up of the following organs: mouth, teeth, tongue salivary glands, pharynx, esophagus, stomach, liver, gallbladder, biliary tract, pancreas, small intestine, large intestine.

The Fart Side: Windbreaks!

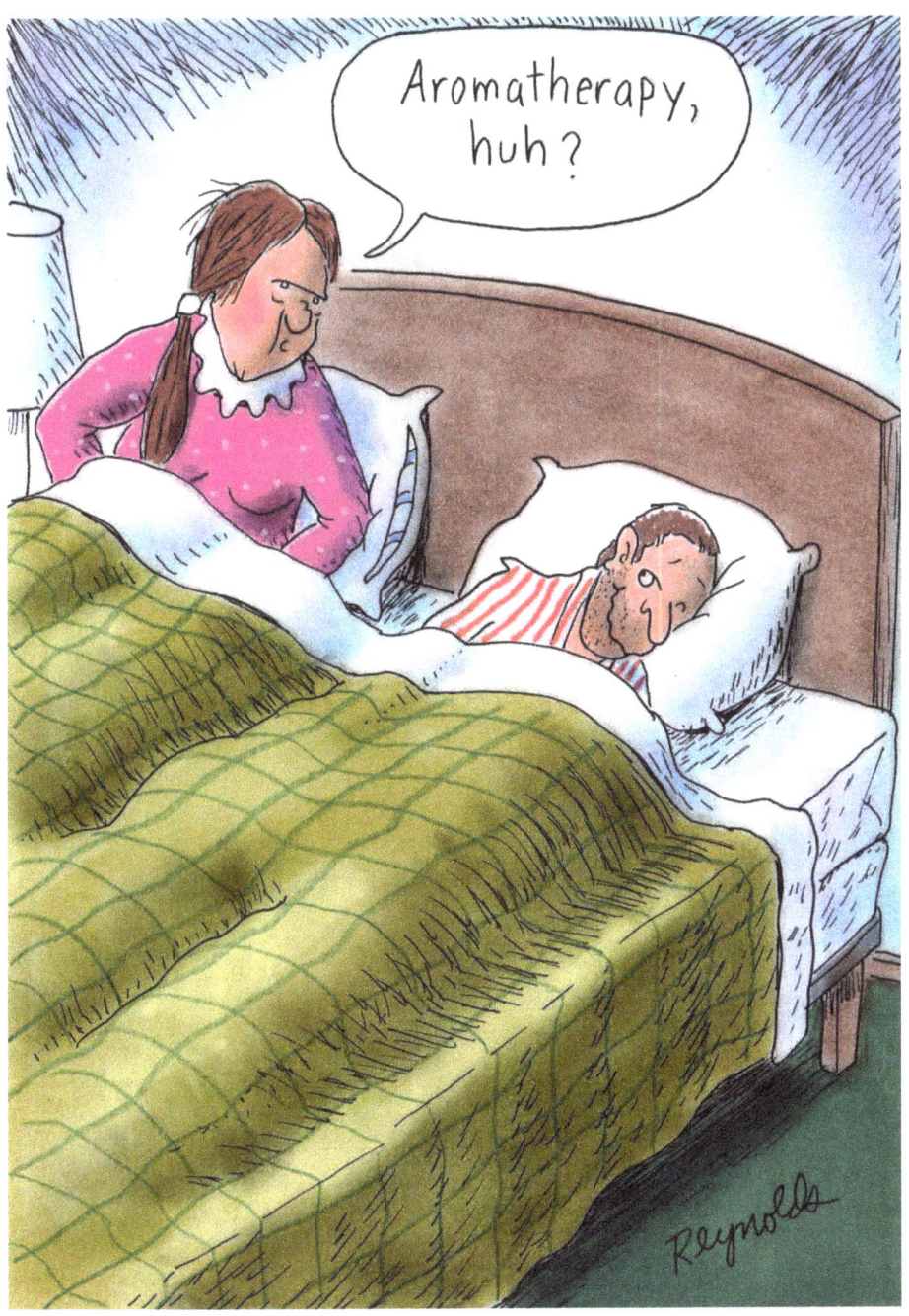

Lactose (from the Latin word lactis milk) is a combination of the simple monosaccharide sugars of galactose and glucose, that is found in milk. Since it has two sugar molecules it is classified as a disaccharide.

Acidophilus milk, and products that contain live Lactobacillus cultures such as yogurts, have reduced lactose content.

Lactose free dairy products are commercially available, as is the milk sugar enzyme supplement lactase. Taken with lactose, it can help with its digestion and processing.

Whey is the liquid remaining after milk is curdled and strained, often for the production of cheese.

The large intestine is approximately five feet (1.5 meters) long, and three inches (7.5 centimeters) in diameter.

The Fart Side: Windbreaks!

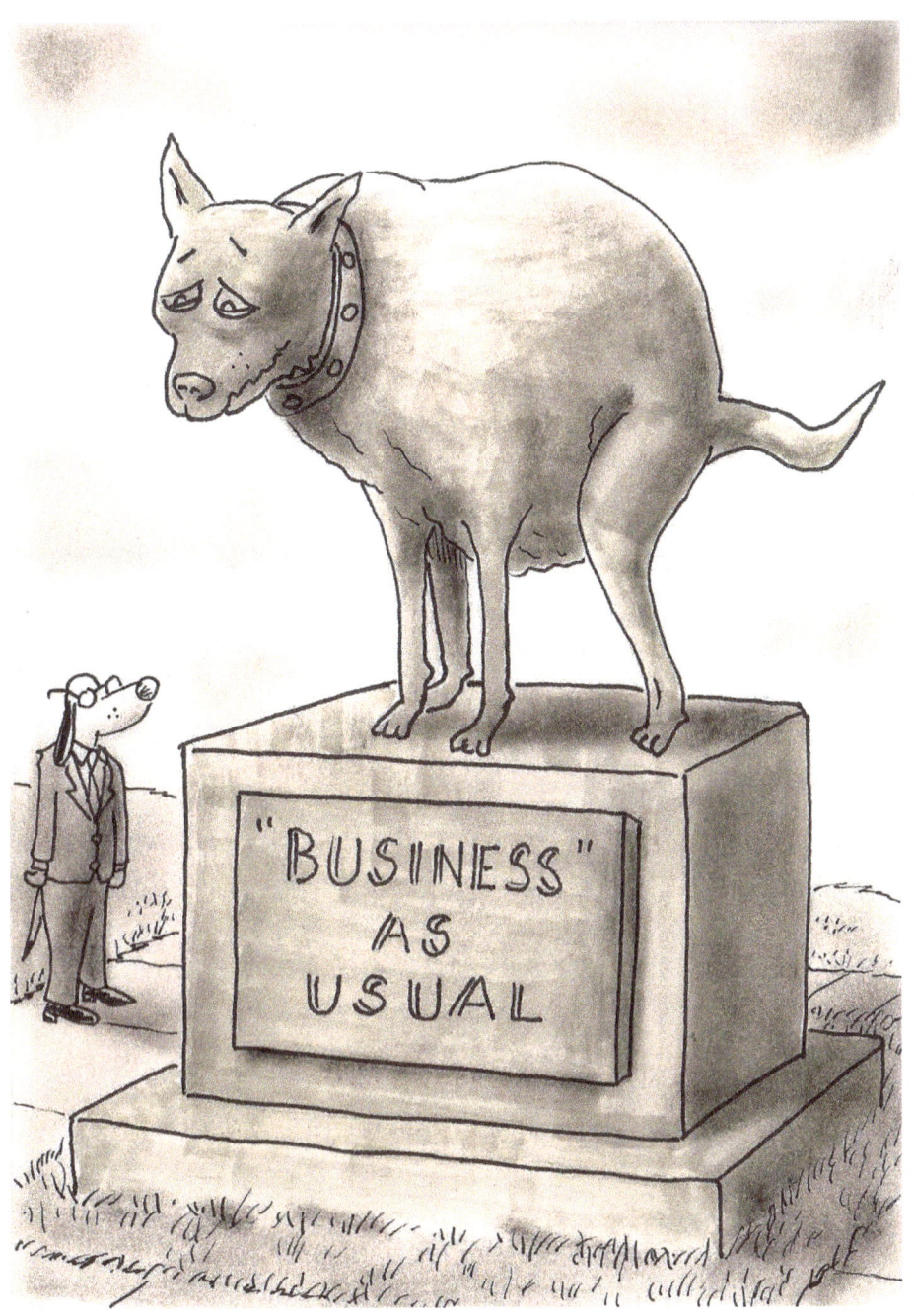

The primary greenhouse gases in the Earth's atmosphere are water vapor, carbon dioxide, methane, nitrous oxide, and ozone.

Clouds, composed of water droplets or ice crystals, contribute to the greenhouse effect.

Venus is a prime example of the planetary temperature consequences of the greenhouse effect.

Lactose is the natural milk sugar often found in cheese, ice cream, and processed foods.

Hard cheeses and yogurts typically have low levels of lactose.

The human stomach directly absorbs water, alcohol, aspirin and non-steroidal anti-inflammatory drugs (NSAIDs).

The Fart Side: Windbreaks!

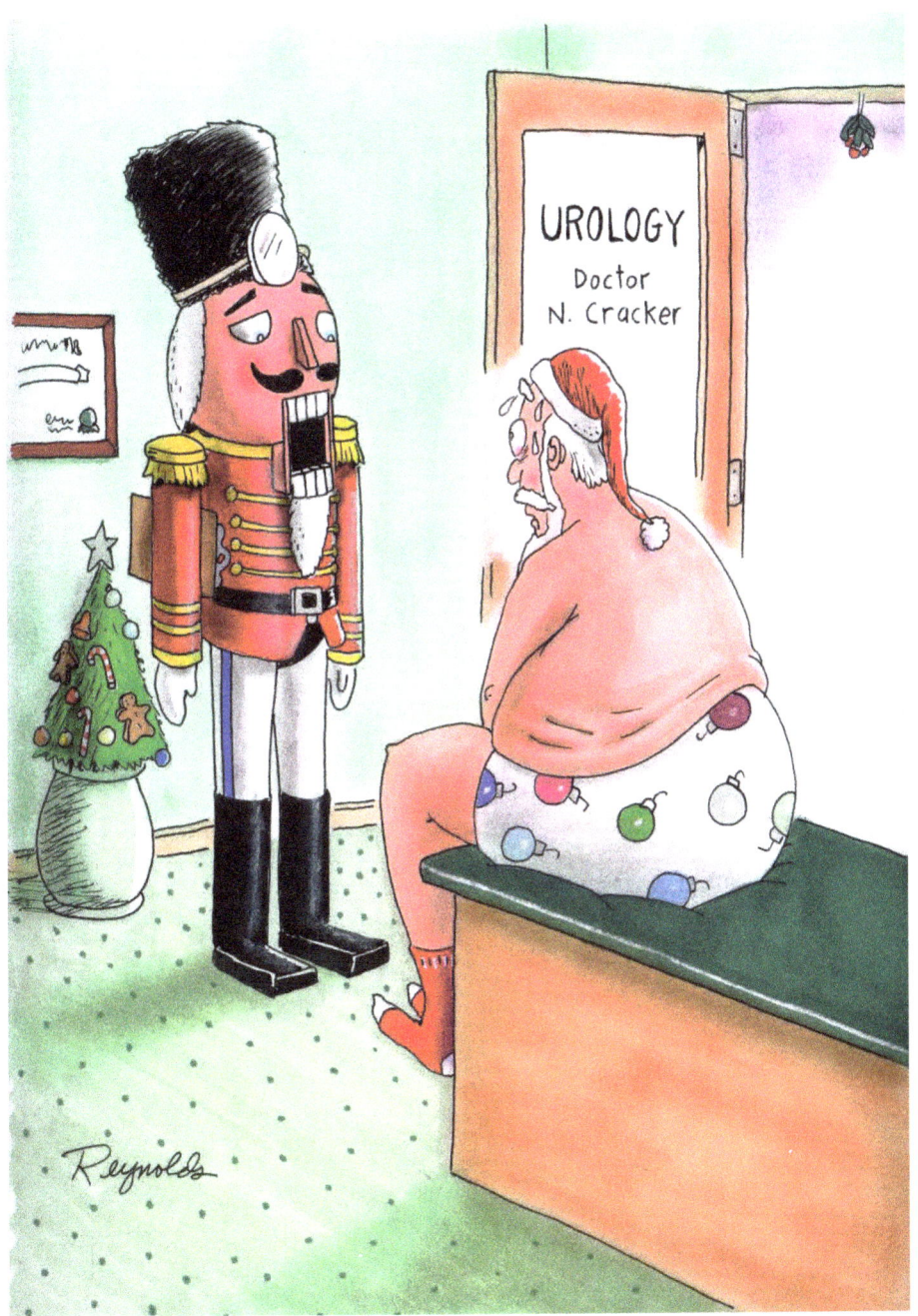

A ruminant (Latin *ruminare* - to chew over again) is a mammal that digests plants in a multi compartment stomach through bacterial fermentation. It regurgitates the semi-digested mass, called cud, and chews it again and repeats the swallow. The process of re-chewing the cud is called rumination.

Bacteria are critical to life on Earth, actively participating in many steps in the nutrient cycles that life depends on. Fixation of nitrogen from the atmosphere is one example.

One cow produces enough manure in one day to generate three-kilowatt hours of electricity, enough to power a one-hundred-watt light bulb for twenty-four hours.

The absorption of nutrients in the gut occurs at microscopic projections of the small intestine lining called villi.

The Fart Side: Windbreaks!

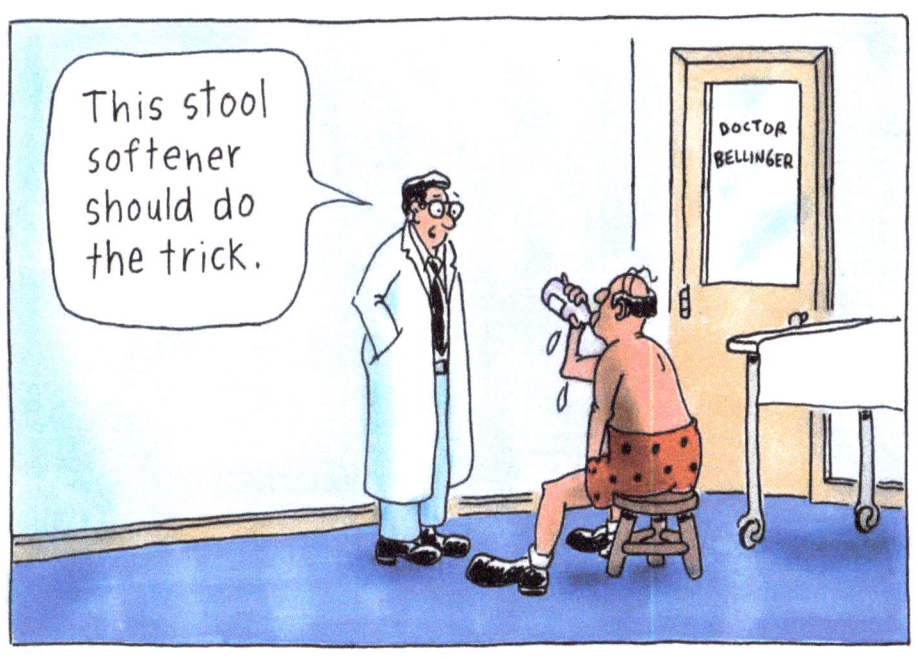

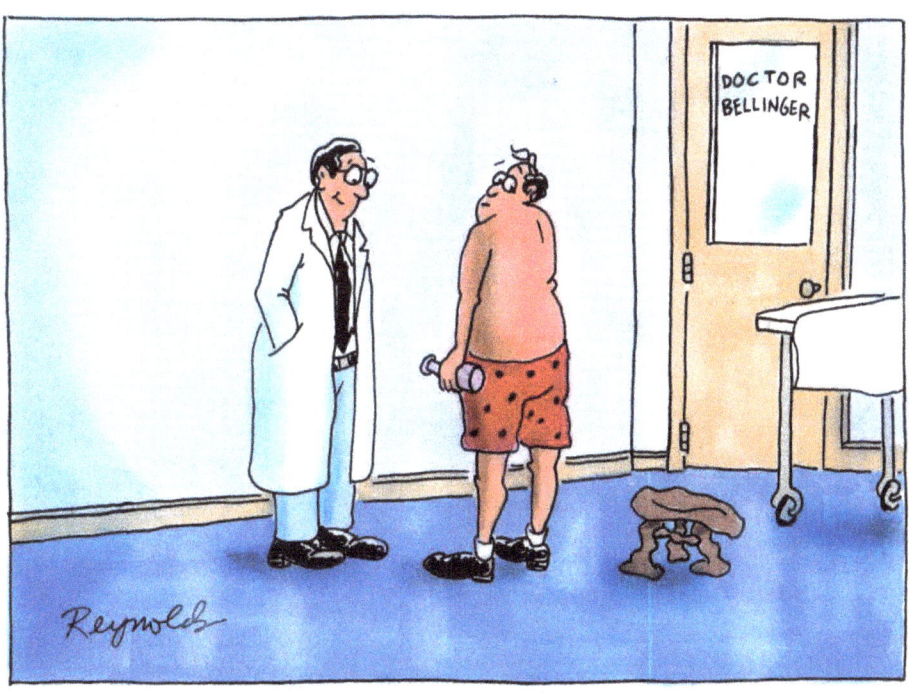

There are more than ten times as many microbial cells in the human microbiome (the microbes that live on and within a human) as there are human cells in the body. Trillions of microbes live on the skin, and over one-hundred trillion within the gut flora.

There are over one hundred species of ruminants, which include both domestic and wild species. Ruminating mammals include cattle, goats, sheep, giraffes, yaks, deer, camels, llamas, and antelope.

Most bacteria have yet to be identified and characterized. The science and study of bacteria is known as bacteriology, and is a branch of microbiology.

The US Department of Agriculture has supported research activities to develop a low fart bean with lower concentrations of the complex sugars that lead to flatulence.

The Fart Side: Windbreaks!

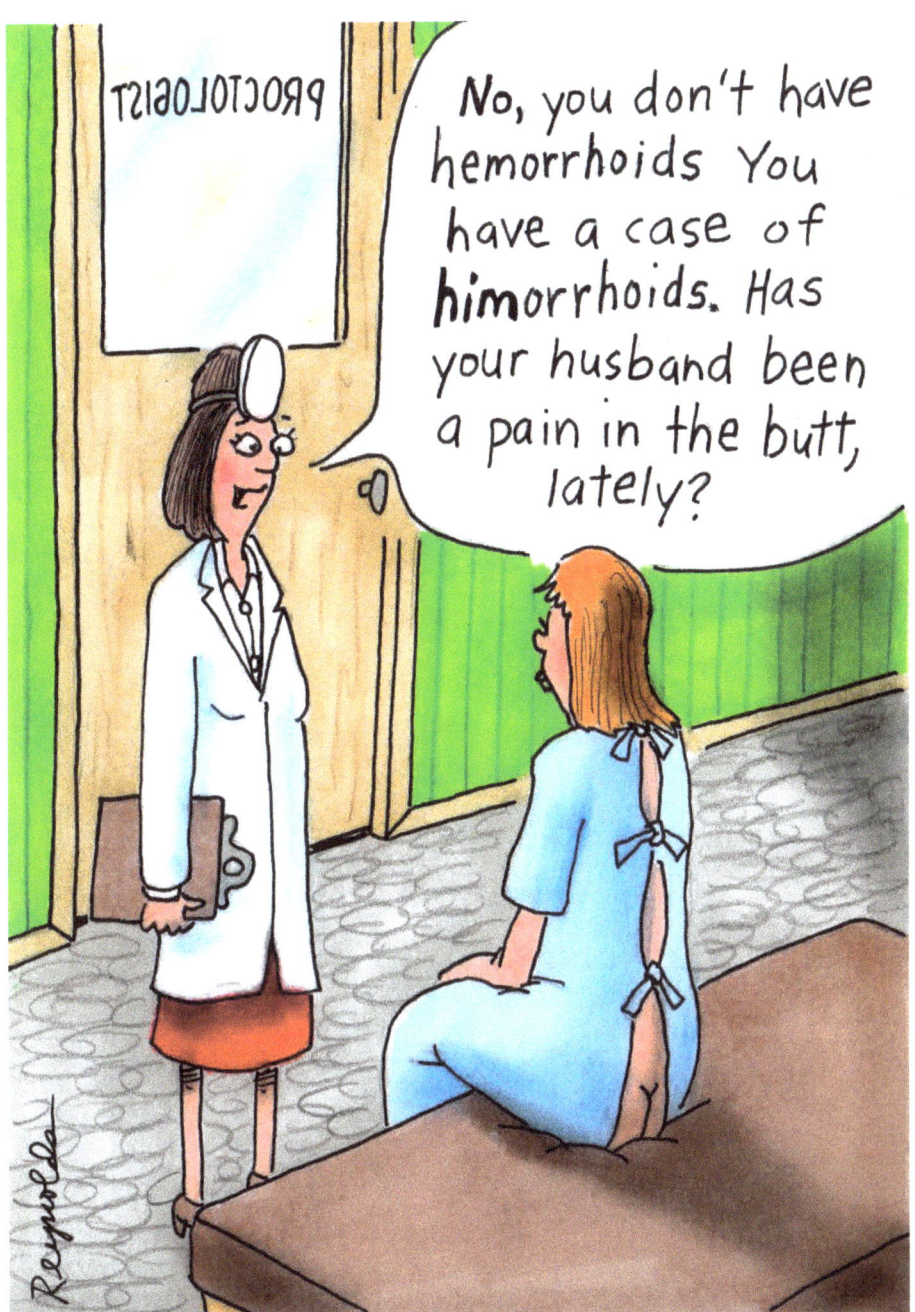

Sternutation is the formal term for a sneeze.

Swimming and motile bacteria frequently move between ten and one hundred body lengths per second. On a relative scale, this makes them at least as fast as fish.

Christian Gottfried Ehrenberg has been credited with being the scientist, who in 1828, introduced the word "bacterium".

The gallbladder is not a vital organ.

Louis Pasteur demonstrated in 1859 that the theory of spontaneous generation was incorrect. He also demonstrated that the fermentation process is caused by the growth of microorganisms, yeasts, and molds.

The human brain can be powerfully influenced by minute quantities of certain plants, foods, microbes, or toxins.

The Fart Side: Windbreaks!

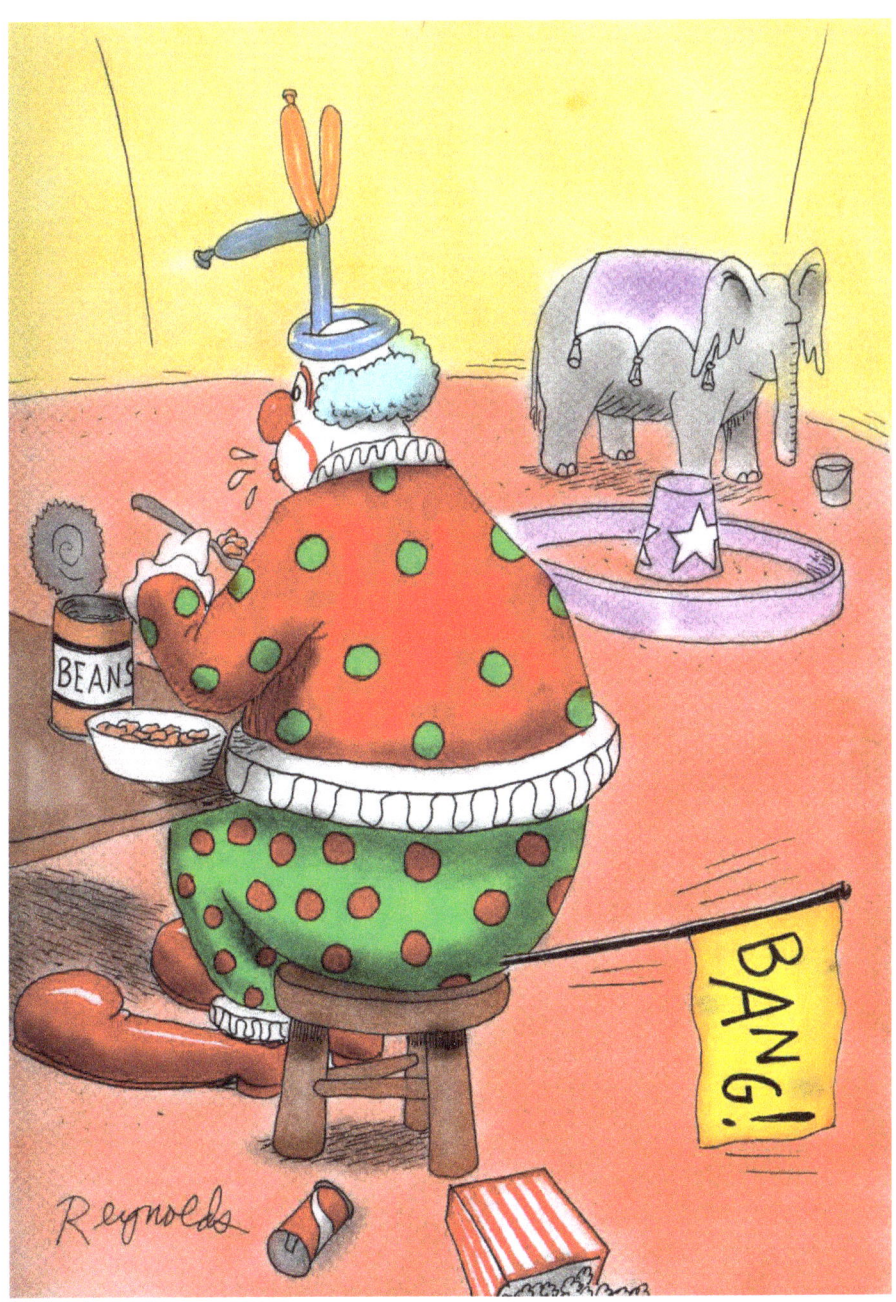

Genetic studies have revealed that fungi are actually more closely related to animals than plants.

Viruses have genes, but they do not have the cellular structure that many define as the basic unit of life.

Viruses do not have an independent metabolism, and must invade a host cell to make new products and replicate.

There are more viruses on Earth than there are stars in the universe. If you stacked every virus end to end, they would stretch over one hundred thousand light years.

Eructation is the formal term for a belch or burp.

An infection can overwhelm a healthy person and lead to death in a matter of hours.

The Fart Side: Windbreaks!

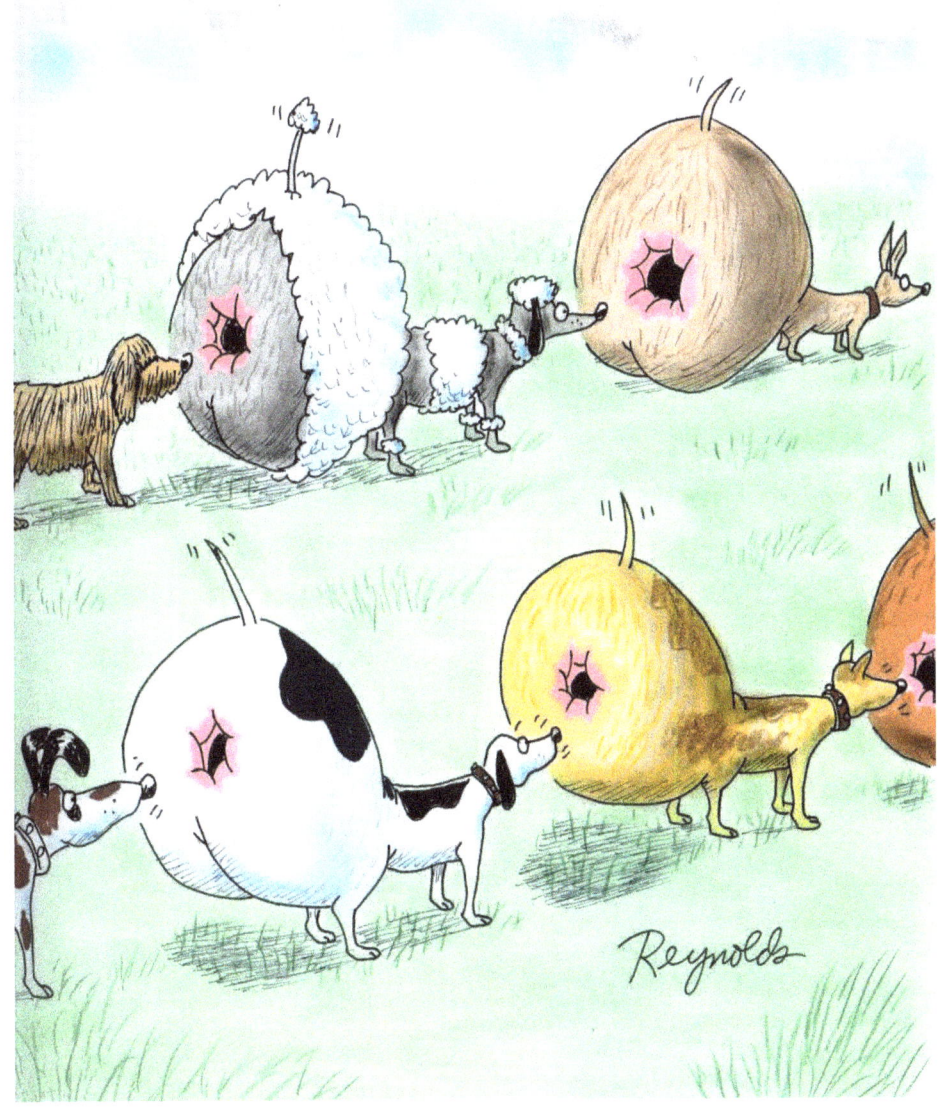

Most people lose the lactase enzyme, that helps to digest the complex milk sugar lactose, after weaning.

The alphabet of the entire genetic code of millions of genes has only five characters.

The most common source of intestinal gas is air swallowing (aerophagia).

The flammable gasses that make lighting a fart dangerous include oxygen, hydrogen, and methane.

Scuba divers are advised to avoid beans before a dive. The gas bubbles in the gut can expand and become painful on ascent because of the decreasing atmospheric pressure.

It is possible to suffocate without any sense of air hunger if deprived of oxygen, as long as carbon dioxide is allowed to be expelled.

The Fart Side: Windbreaks!

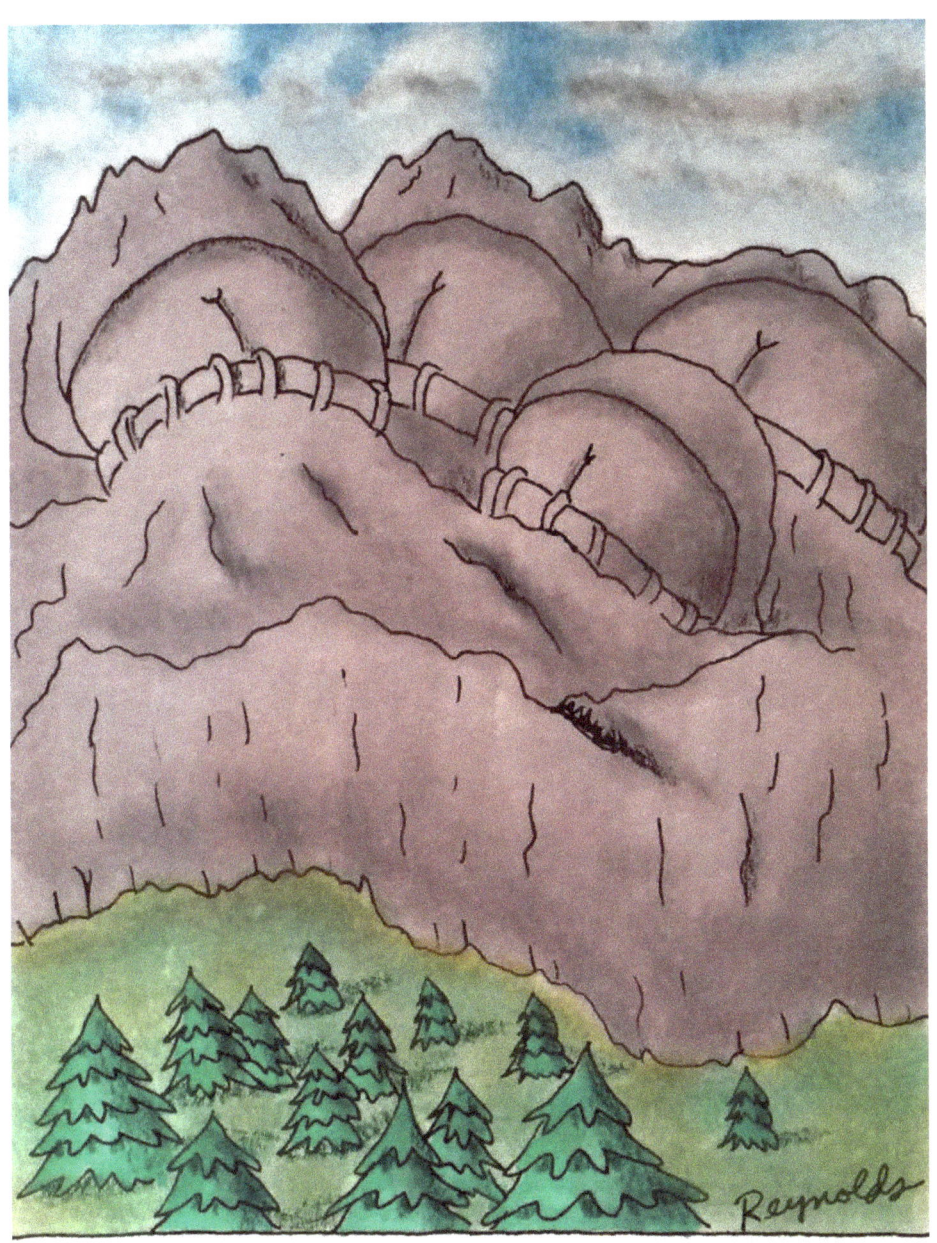

Women either fart somewhat less often than men, or more likely, just deny it more often.

The enzymes produced by the digestive organs are commercially available. They are helpful as supplements if needed.

The primary purpose of the stomach is to mix food with acid and enzymes.

Reflex and heartburn increases the risk of esophagus cancer.

Constipation does not increase the risk of colon cancer.

The human and chimpanzee genome is 98.5% identical.

Most the products sold to consumers in the forty billion dollars a year probiotic market has no scientific proof of providing a benefit.

The Fart Side: Windbreaks!

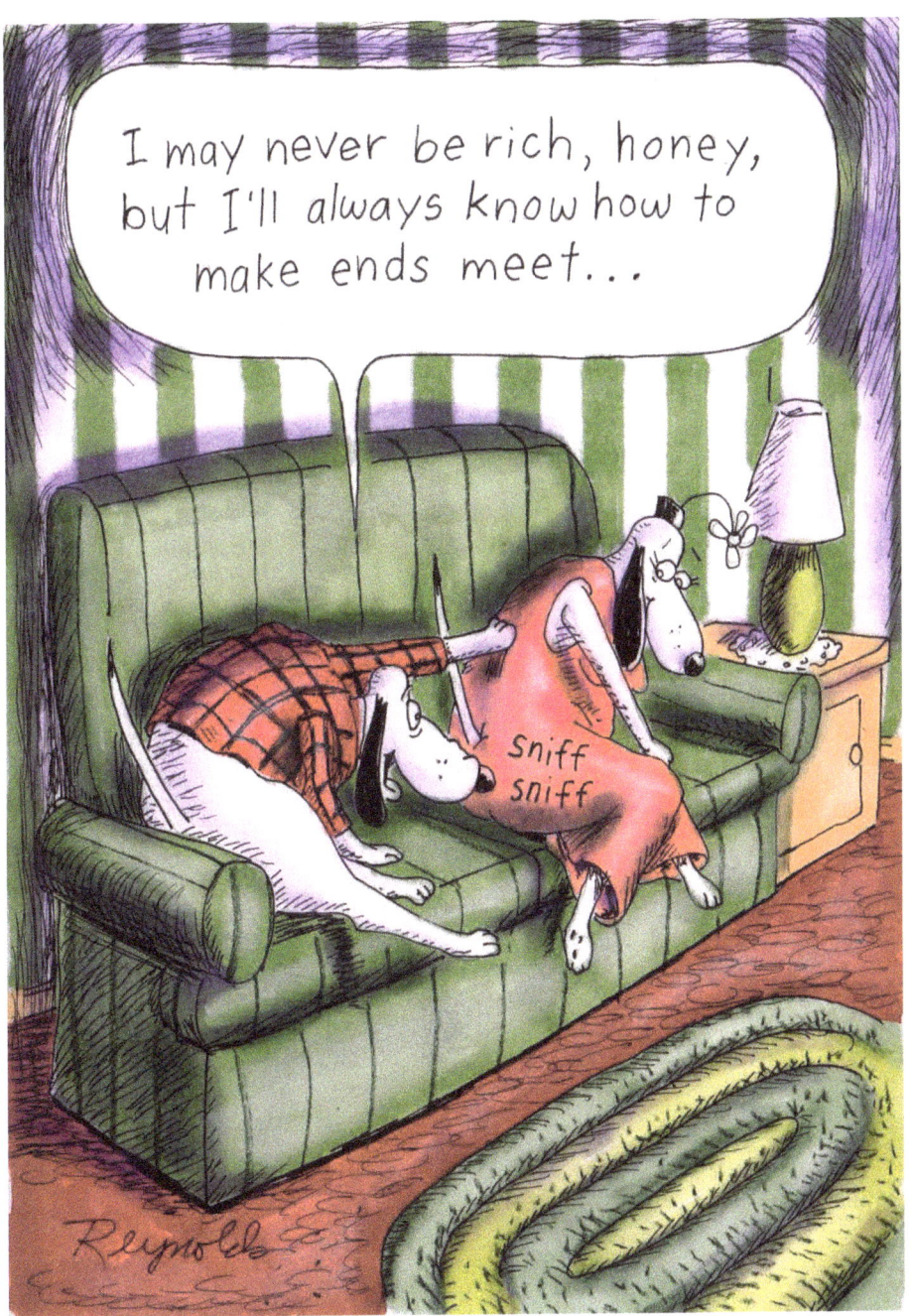

Thirty percent of the genes of humans and microbes are identical.

The vast majority of the microbes present are a healthy part of the gut microbiome.

The neurotransmitter serotonin is found in much higher concentrations in the gut, than in the brain.

The brain and gut are in constant communication.

The vagus nerve has over eighty percent of the messaging traffic going from the gut to the brain.

The aroma of a fart can be an indicator of intestinal health.

Many pharmaceuticals contain lactose as a filler, that is rarely mentioned on the label despite lactose intolerance being very common.

The Fart Side: Windbreaks!

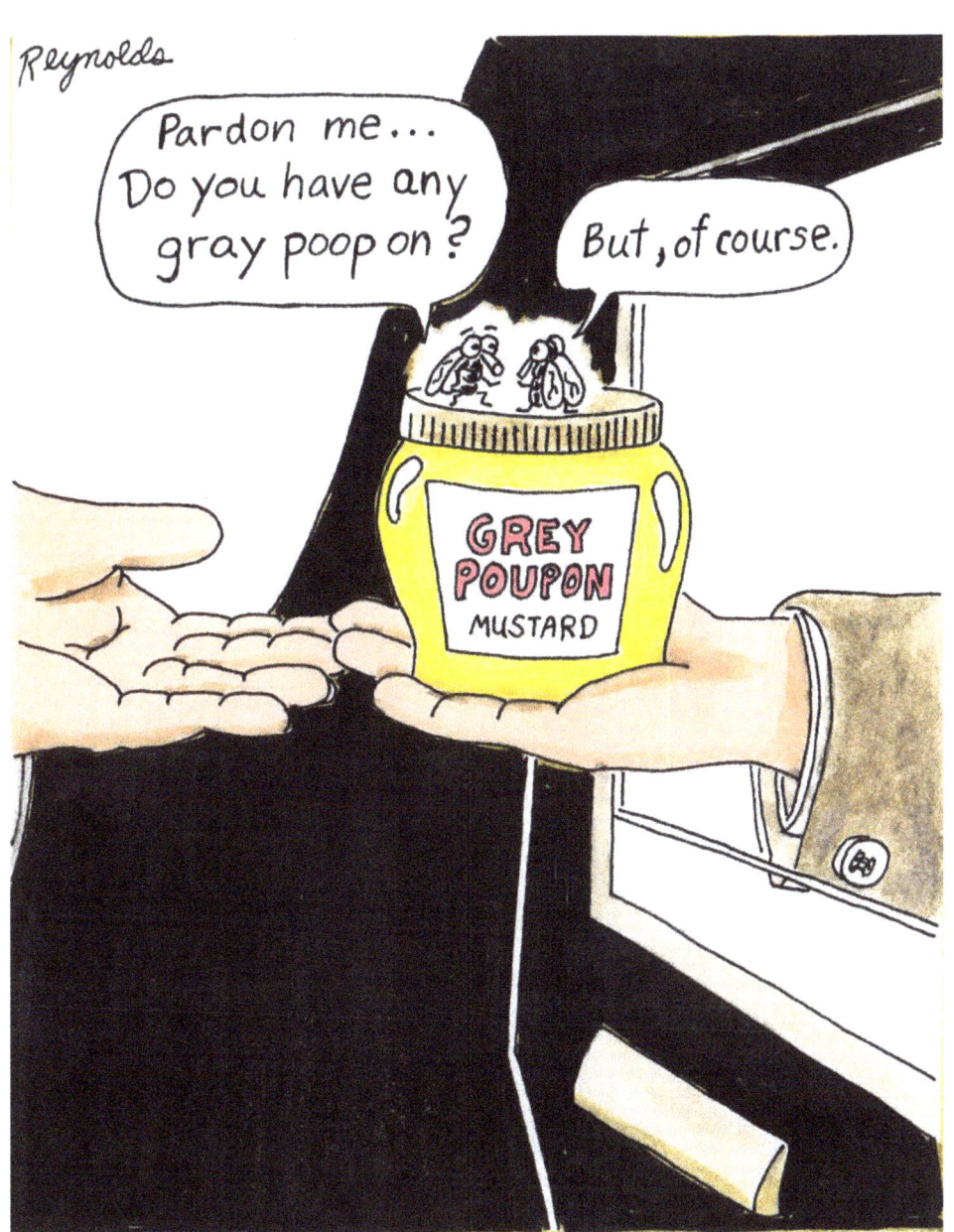

Fly Commercials

Over ninety-nine percent of the gas passed in a fart is odorless.

Beer poured in Denver will have a larger head of bubbles than the same beer poured in Seattle, due to altitude.

A hiccup is caused by the involuntary contraction of the diaphragm.

Carbon dioxide gas dissolved in water produces carbonic acid.

Nitrogen bubbles in a beverage are smaller and longer lasting than carbon dioxide bubbles.

Half of the bodies supply of the major neurotransmitter dopamine is in the gut, and the other half is in the brain.

More than four hundred thousand people die in US hospitals each year because of preventable errors.

The Fart Side: Windbreaks!

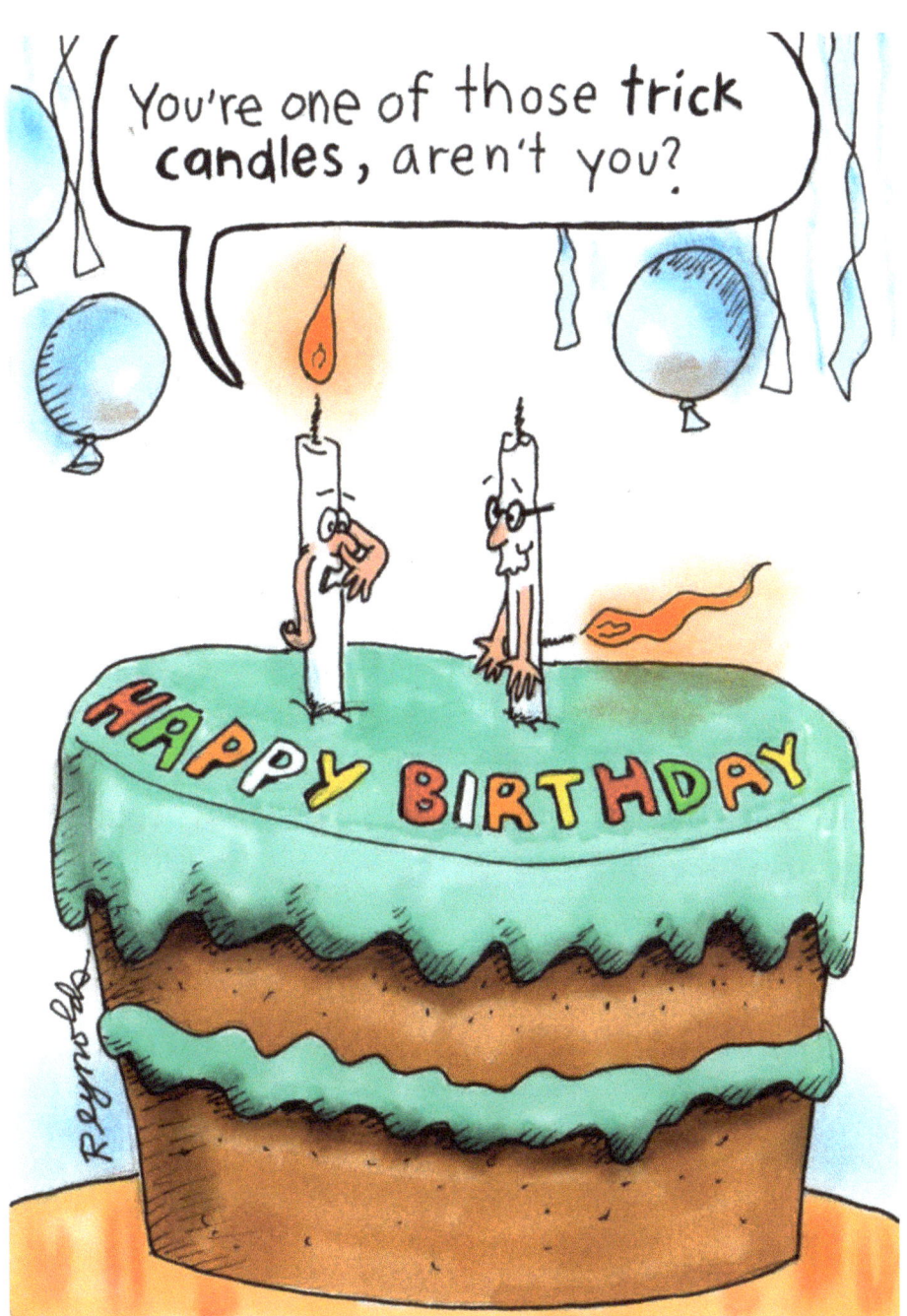

Hemorrhoids are part of normal anatomy, and have an important function in maintaining continence.

The neurological disorders Parkinson Disease and Alzheimer Disease are believed to originate in the gut with the gut microbiome.

The number of species of microbes in the human microbiome is believed to be in the tens of thousands.

The number of genes in the human body is one percent human, and ninety-nine percent from microbes.

The oldest and most numerous organisms on Earth, called Archaea, were discovered less than fifty years ago.

Ice cream is often forty percent air by volume, and contributes to intestinal gas.

The Fart Side: Windbreaks!

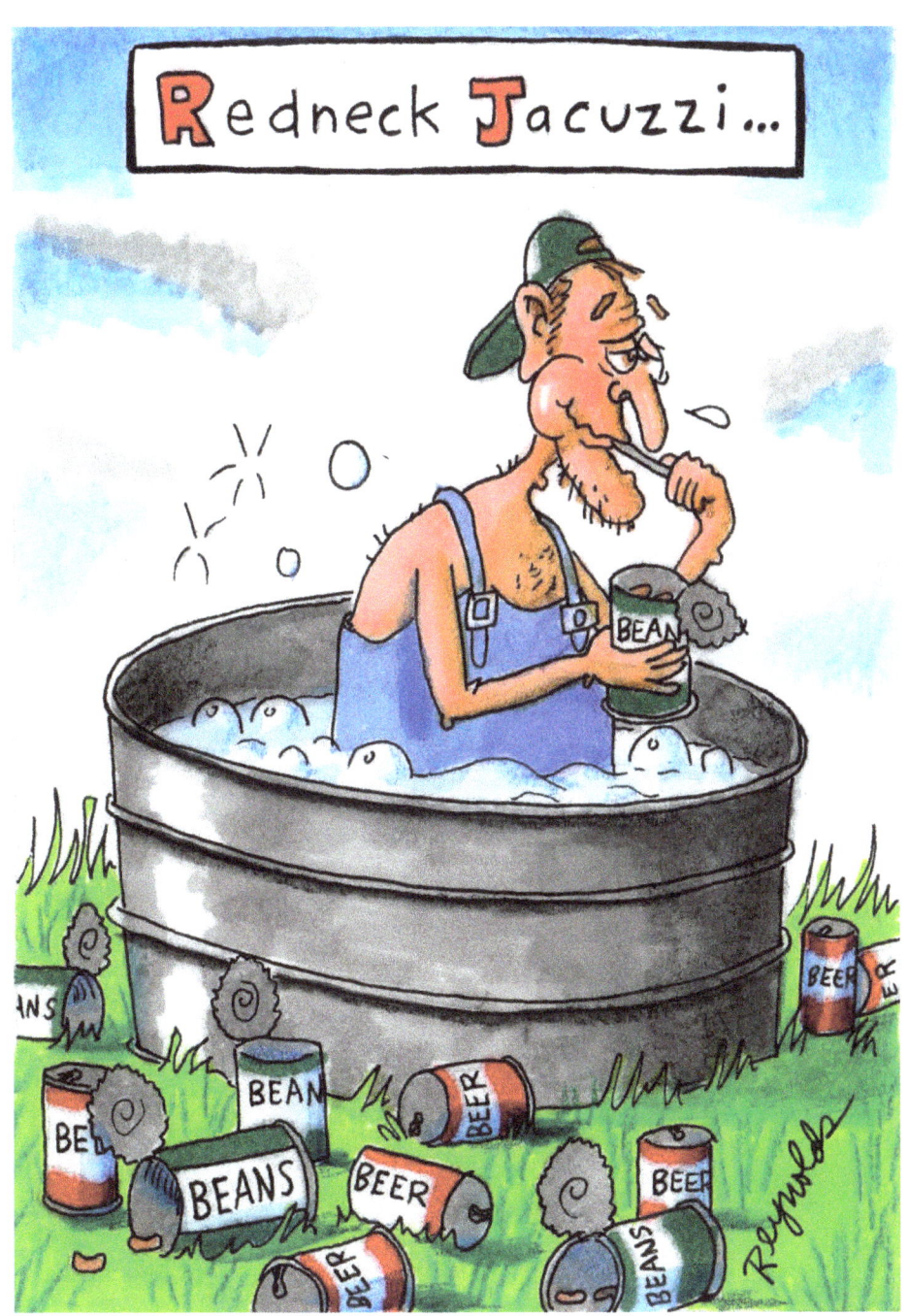

Most pharmaceuticals marketed in the US do not have proven effectiveness.

Tussis is the formal term for a cough.

Meteorism is an older British term for farting.

Aspirin in children and young adults can be dangerous if they have a viral infection.

Mastication is the formal term for chewing.

Poor fitting dentures can contribute to intestinal gas.

The enzyme amylase in saliva converts the amylose starch of a potato chip into the sweeter taste of starch sugars in a matter of minutes.

Enzyme supplements to reduce gas from beans and legumes can be effective.

The Fart Side: Windbreaks!

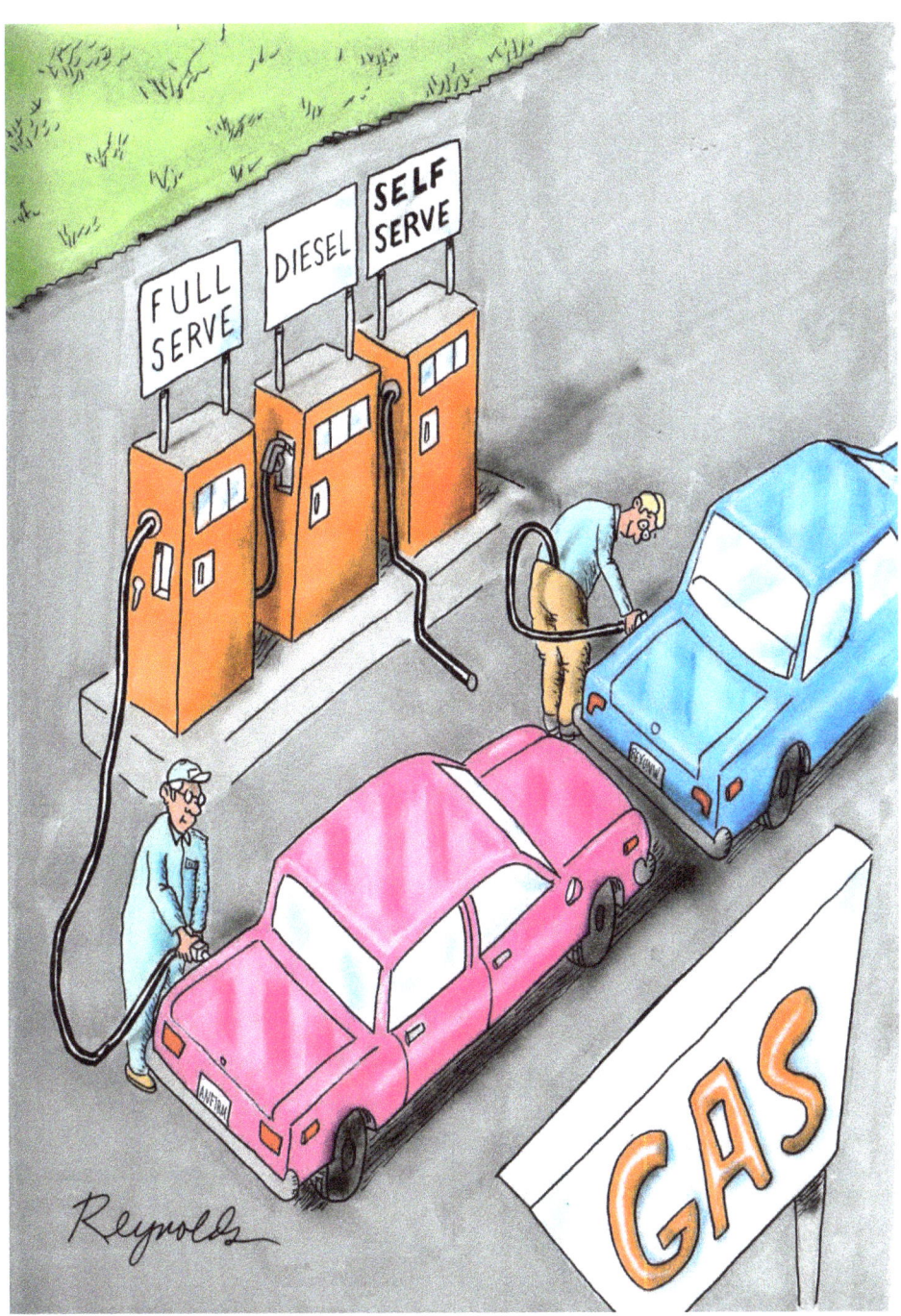

Growing evidence suggests that obesity and diabetes mellitus is powerfully influenced by the microbes that live within the gut.

Many liters of carbon dioxide gas are produced when stomach acid is neutralized by pancreatic secretions of sodium bicarbonate. The carbon dioxide is rapidly absorbed into the bloodstream and exhaled by the lungs.

One gram (one ounce contains more than twenty-eight grams) of activated charcoal has a surface area greater than five hundred square meters (one thousand five hundred square feet).

Sipping smaller volumes increases the amount of air swallowed (aerophagia).

The risk of dying from colon cancer can be greatly reduced by routine screening tests.

The Fart Side: Windbreaks!

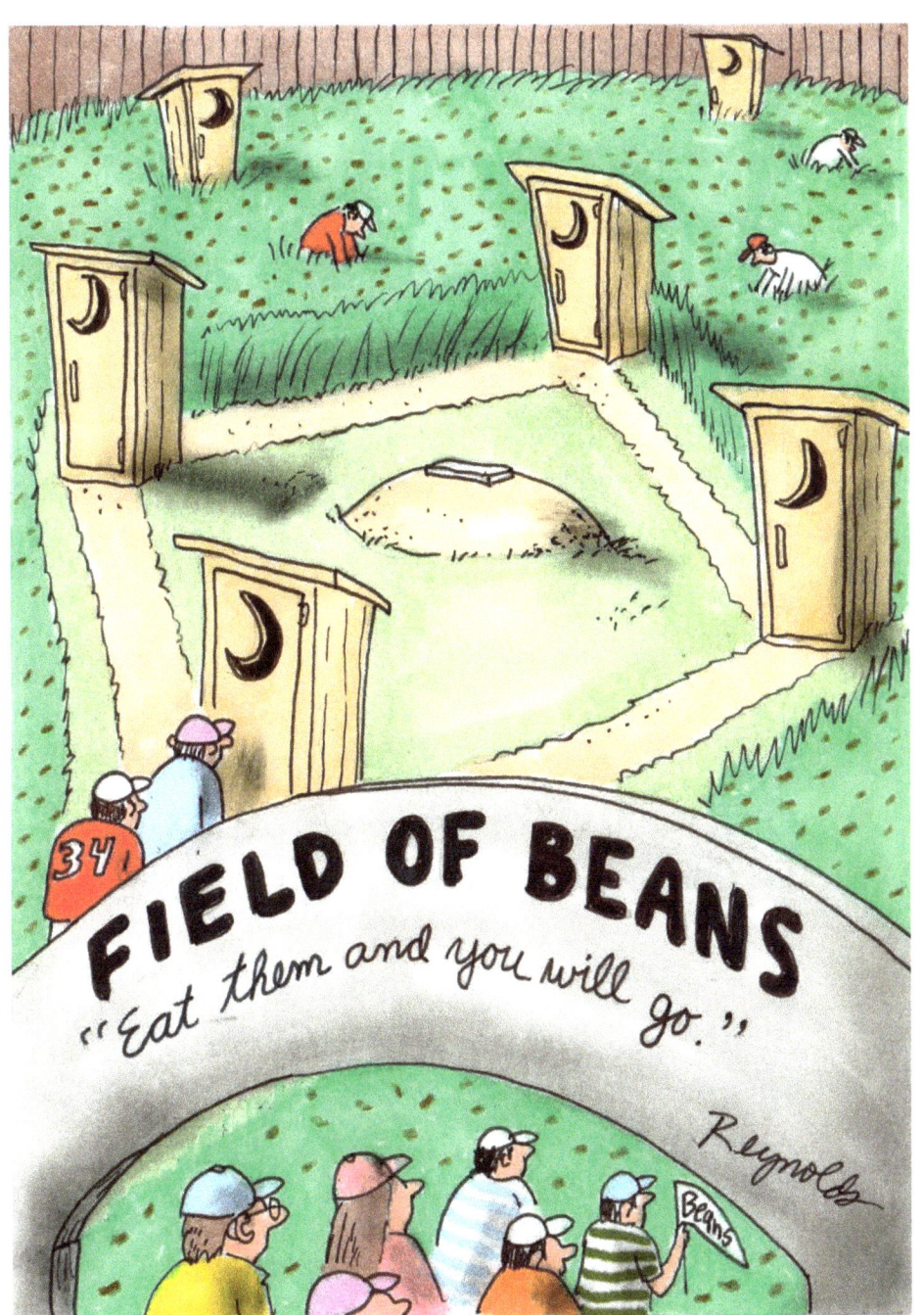

Carbon dioxide comprises less than one percent of the composition of air.

Air is seventy-eight percent nitrogen, which is a gas that is very poorly absorbed by the gut.

The average person swallows two thousand times per day, and each swallow includes five milliliters (one teaspoon) of air.

The ten liters of air swallowed every day is seventy- eight percent nitrogen, which since it is not well absorbed, must be released as a burp or as a fart.

A typical one-liter container of a carbonated beverage has one liter of fluid, and an additional nearly three liters of carbon dioxide gas in solution.

Most the human population harbors parasites.

The Fart Side: Windbreaks!

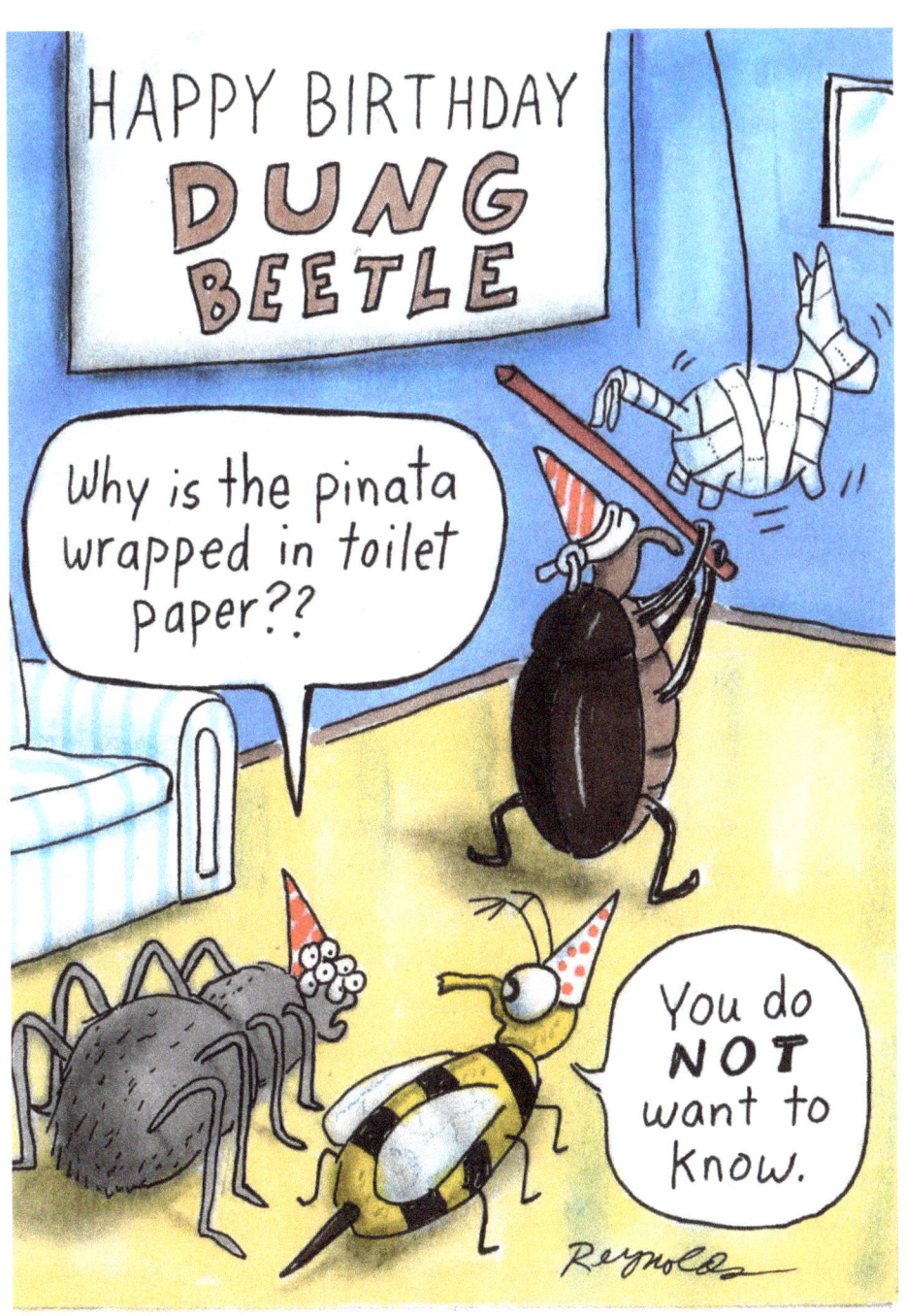

Your toothbrush is not safe from fecal contamination, even if the counter where it is kept is twenty feet away from the toilet.

The average person swallows every thirty seconds while awake, and every five minutes while asleep.

Most people fart while they sleep, and occasionally it is loud or aromatic enough to awake themselves (or a sleeping partner).

Carbonated beverages outsell dairy products by a ratio of four to one in the United States.

Carbon dioxide in solution can convert water to carbonic acid, which can damage the enamel of teeth leading to tooth decay.

More than twenty-five billion rolls of toilet paper are sold every year in the U.S.

The Fart Side: Windbreaks!

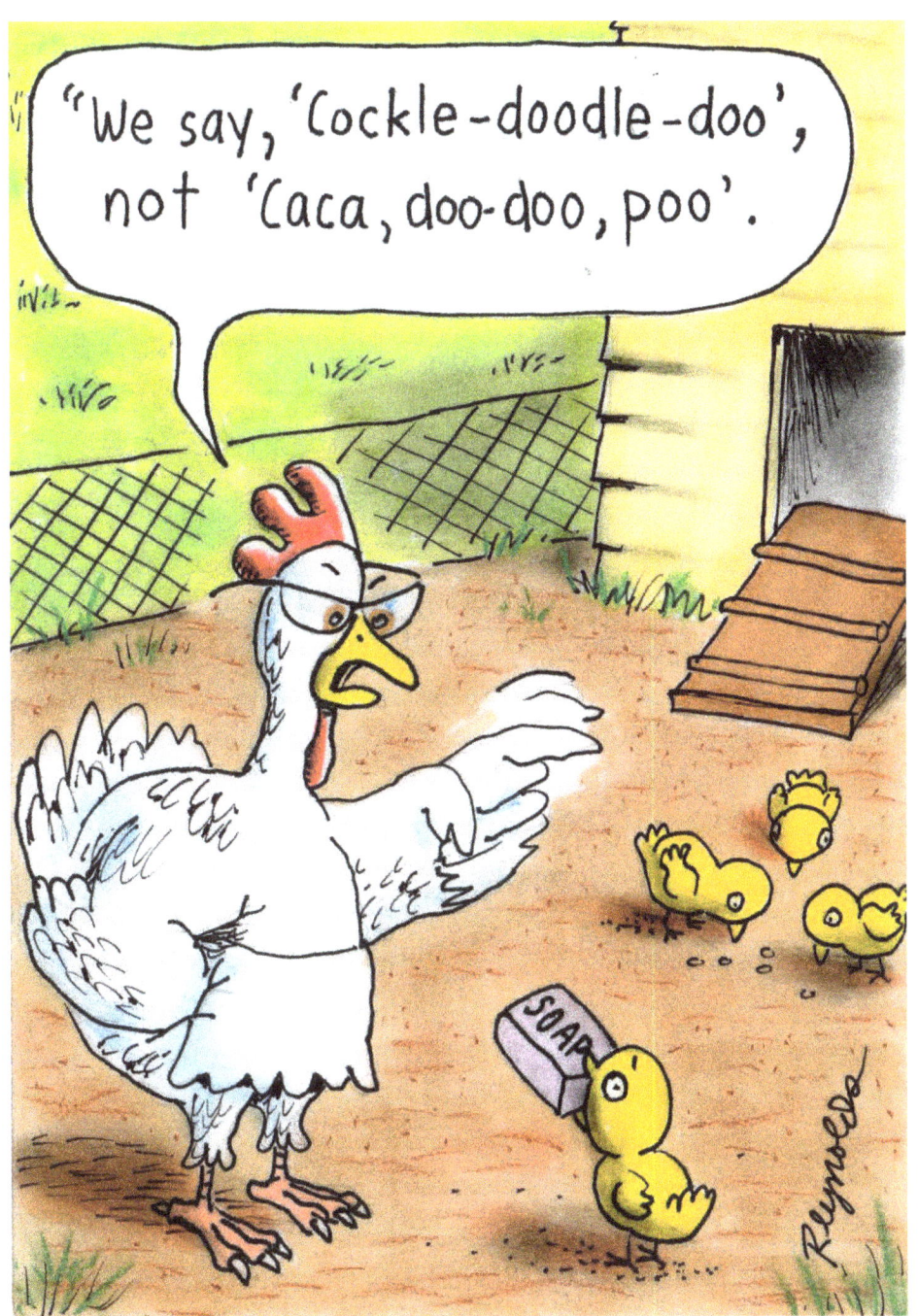

The human stomach can hold approximately 1.6 quarts (1.5 liters) of material when full, and as little as 1.6 fluid ounces (50 milliliters) when empty.

Pilots flying at altitudes over thirty thousand feet in unpressurized aircraft often experience severe abdominal pain from intestinal gas distension. This arises because of the much lower atmospheric pressure, resulting in expansion of gastrointestinal gas.

In space travel the toilet seat has specialized restraints. These are needed so that a fart does not propel the astronaut off the seat due to weightlessness.

While living at high altitude, such as Denver or Mexico City, intestinal gas volume is significantly increased because of the lower atmospheric pressure.

The Fart Side: Windbreaks!

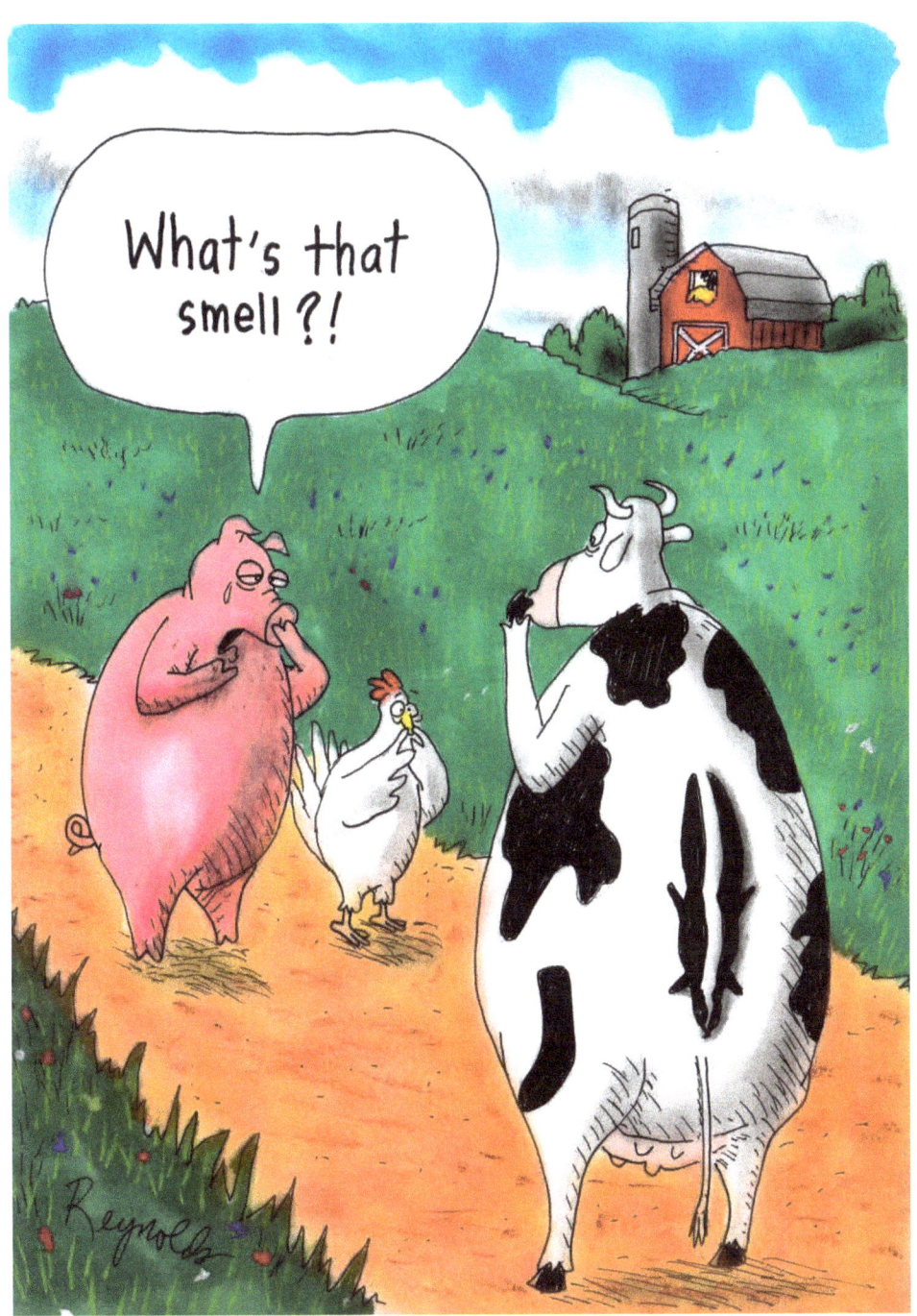

Without saliva, you would not be able to taste, speak, chew, or swallow. It serves as an important lubricant and protectant.

The esophagus is approximately ten inches (25 centimeters) long.

Carbonation using carbon dioxide gas creates larger bubbles and a less longer lasting foam head than nitrogenation using nitrogen gas.

Toilet paper was used in ancient China. Before 1900 hardwood pulp was often used in toilet paper and the possibility of having wood splinters after wiping was an unpleasant consequence.

Nearly thirty thousand trees a day are converted into toilet paper.

Having a bowel movement is easier if sitting on a toilet where the feet can reach the ground to aid in the passage of stool.

The Fart Side: Windbreaks!

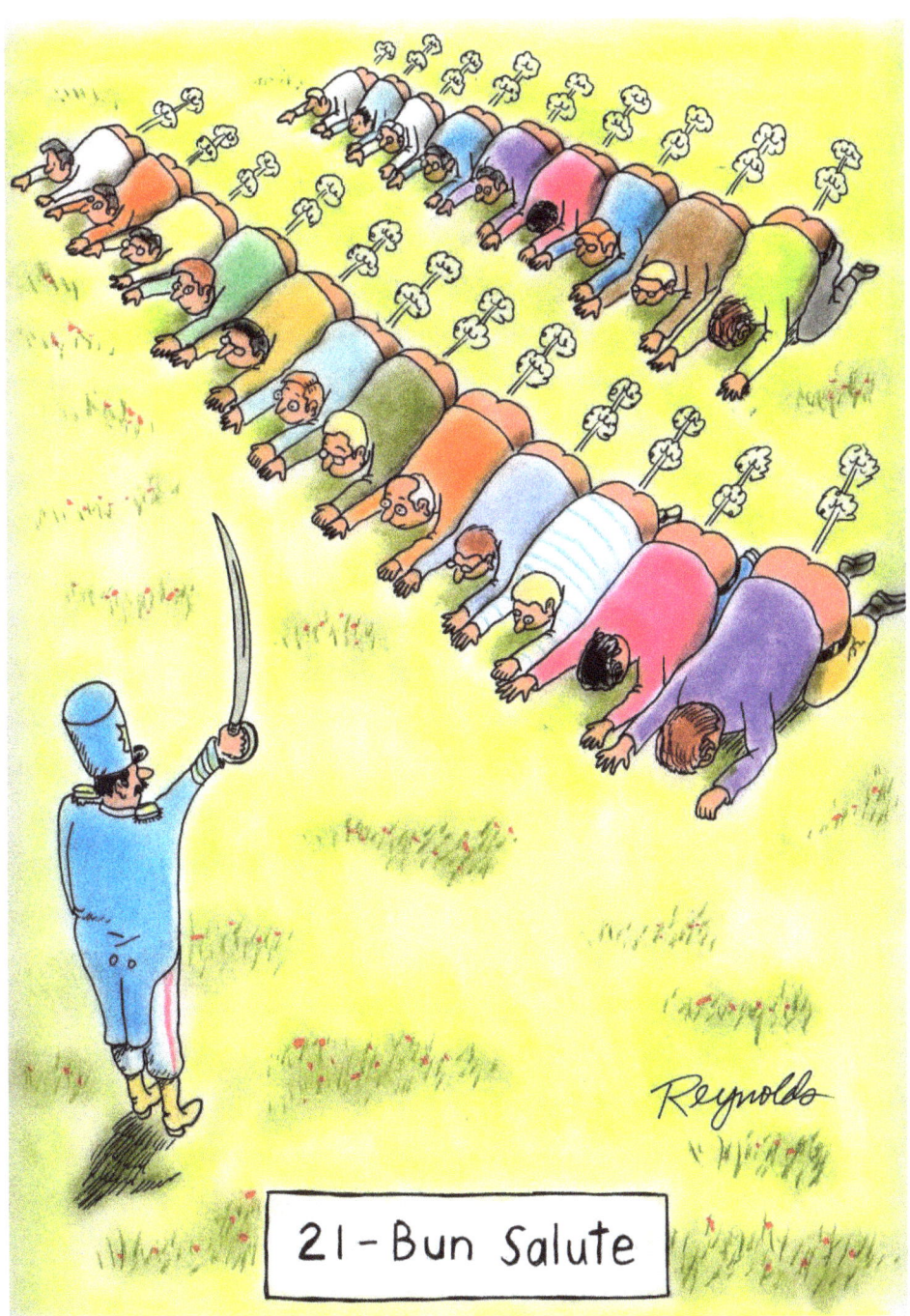

Using toilet paper for anal cleansing is not hygienic, using cleansing water from a bidet is preferable.

In the U.S., more than fifty miles (eighty kilometers) of toilet paper is produced every second of the day and night, throughout the year.

The average person goes to the toilet two thousand five-hundred times per year, and spends a total of three years of their lifetime sitting on the toilet.

One third of Americans flush while still sitting on the toilet. This is actually very dangerous on aircraft and cruise ships with a vacuum flush system. The powerful vacuum flush can lead to severe internal injuries, if a tight seal occurs with sitting.

There are forty thousand injuries a year while sitting on the toilet seat.

The Fart Side: Windbreaks!

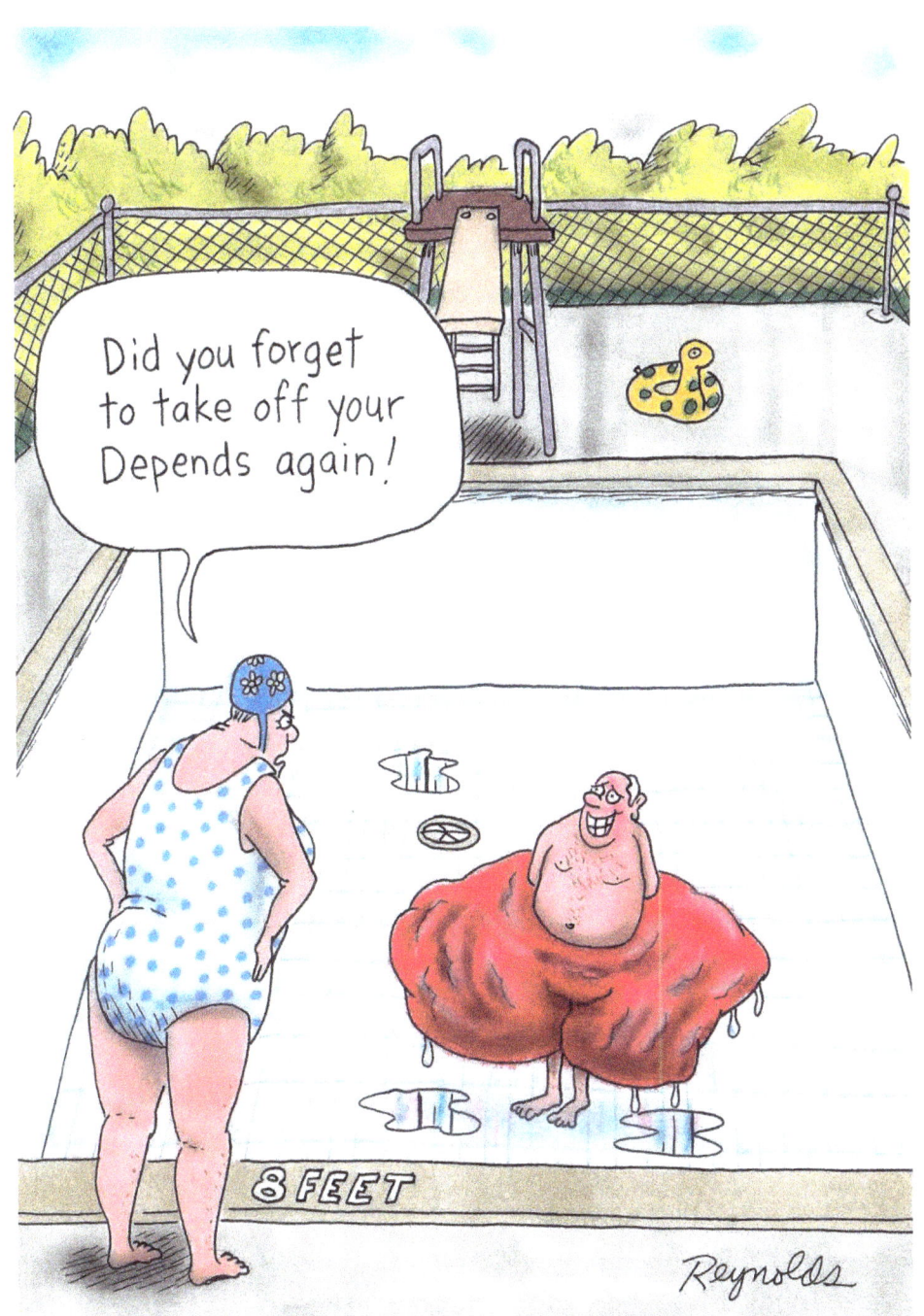

The typical toilet flush creates an aerosolized mist containing fecal contaminants that spreads over a four hundred square foot range. Keep the toilet lid down when flushing.

The tissue of the gut actively secretes and releases hormones that help to regulate the digestive process.

Toilet seats in most U.S. homes have lower microbial populations than kitchen faucets and refrigerator handles. They are simply being cleaned more often.

After nearly ten years, a mattress will double in weight with the feces of mites and dust accumulating.

Singultus is the medical term for hiccups.

The average human eats about 1,200 pounds (500kg) of food per year.

The Fart Side: Windbreaks!

The Latest Version of Smart Phones For Dads....

"This one comes with an app that blames it on the dog."

PHHBBRRT!

"FART" PHONES

Reynolds

The average person produces 1.8 quarts (1.7 liters) of saliva (spit) is each day.

Saliva contains digestive enzymes, mucus, and water.

There are on average one hundred times more bacterial contaminants on restaurant menus than on restaurant toilet seats. The toilet seats are cleaned regularly, while the menus are not.

The kitchen sponge is nearly always the most heavily contaminated item in the house. With ten million microbes per square inch, the kitchen sponge is nearly a quarter of a million times dirtier than a toilet seat.

Humans shed one and one half million skin cells per hour.

A rare turtle in Australia can breathe through its cloaca anus equivalent.

The Fart Side: Windbreaks!

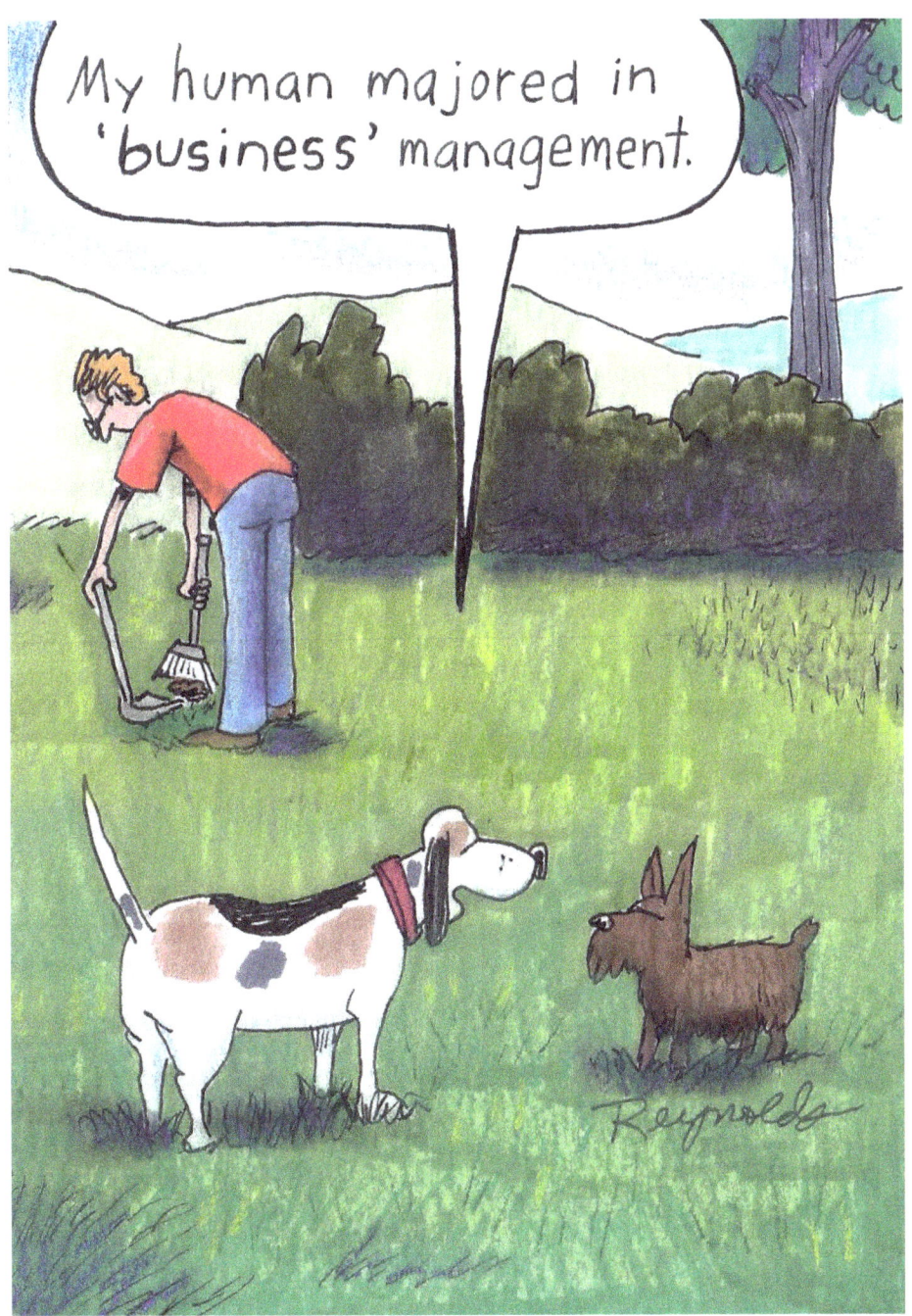

Horses cannot vomit (throw up) because the esophagus in horses has only a one-way direction of movement.

Going up in an elevator in a high-rise building can cause an increase in farting. This is because intestinal gasses expand as the atmospheric pressure decreases with ascent, and reaching higher altitudes.

Digestive enzymes accelerate metabolic activities so that they take place millions of times faster than they would if the enzyme were absent.

Certain insects can walk on water, because of the physical property of surface tension.

Canaries were used as an indicator for safety in coal mines. The sudden death of the canary serving as a warning of the presence of dangerous methane.

The Fart Side: Windbreaks!

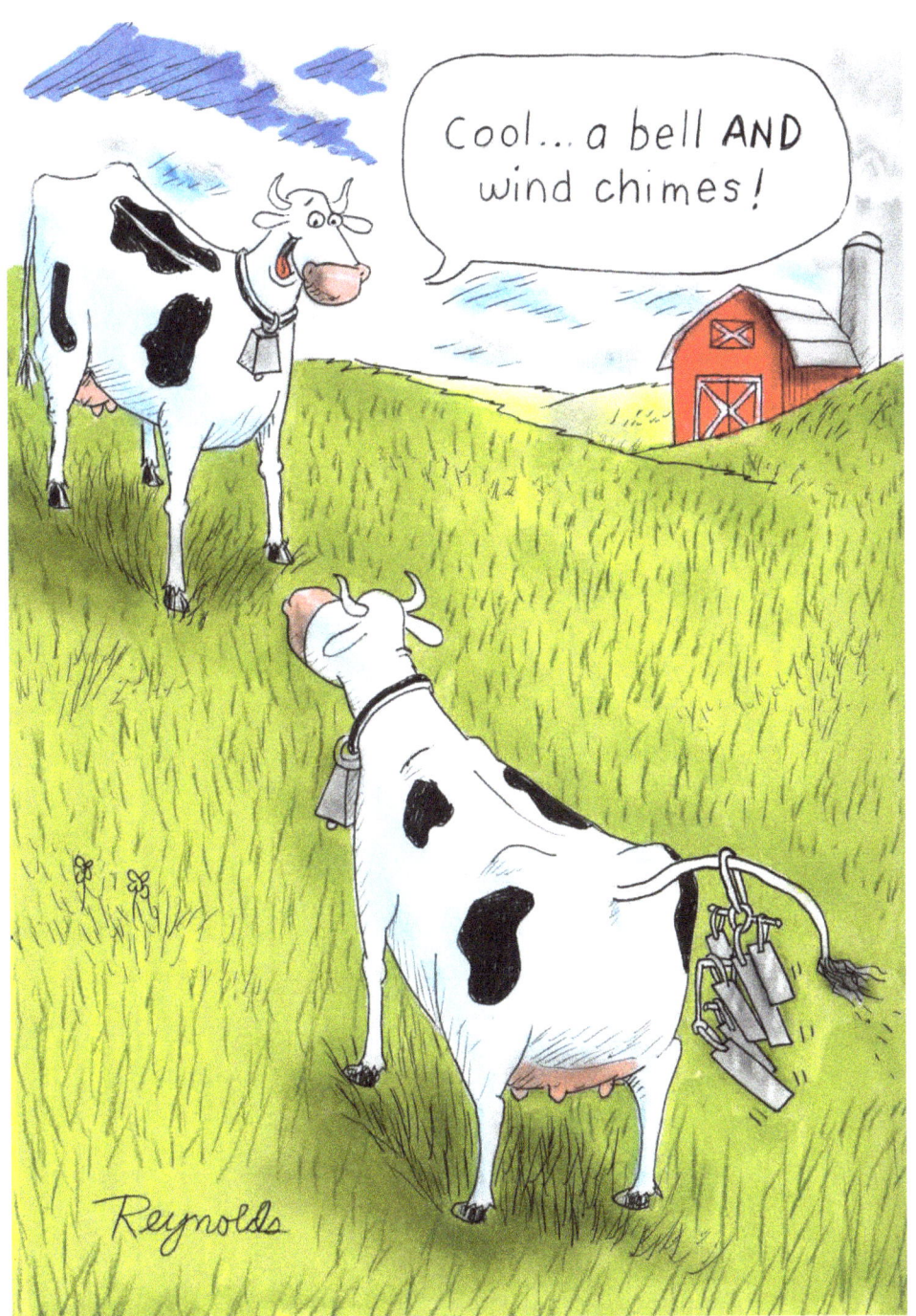

Muscles contract in synchronized waves called peristalsis to move the food in the esophagus (foodpipe/gullet) to the stomach. This means that food would get to a person's stomach even if they were swallowing upside down while standing on their head (not a recommended activity).

Carbon dioxide gas is heavier than air.

Surface tension is the physical principle that causes water to form droplets, soap to create bubbles, and beads of liquids to form on a flat surface.

A carbonated beverage in a plastic bottle will lose its carbonation, and go flat, after just a few months. The carbon dioxide leaves the solution and diffuses through the plastic with time.

Worldwide two million people die each year from diarrhea.

The Fart Side: Windbreaks!

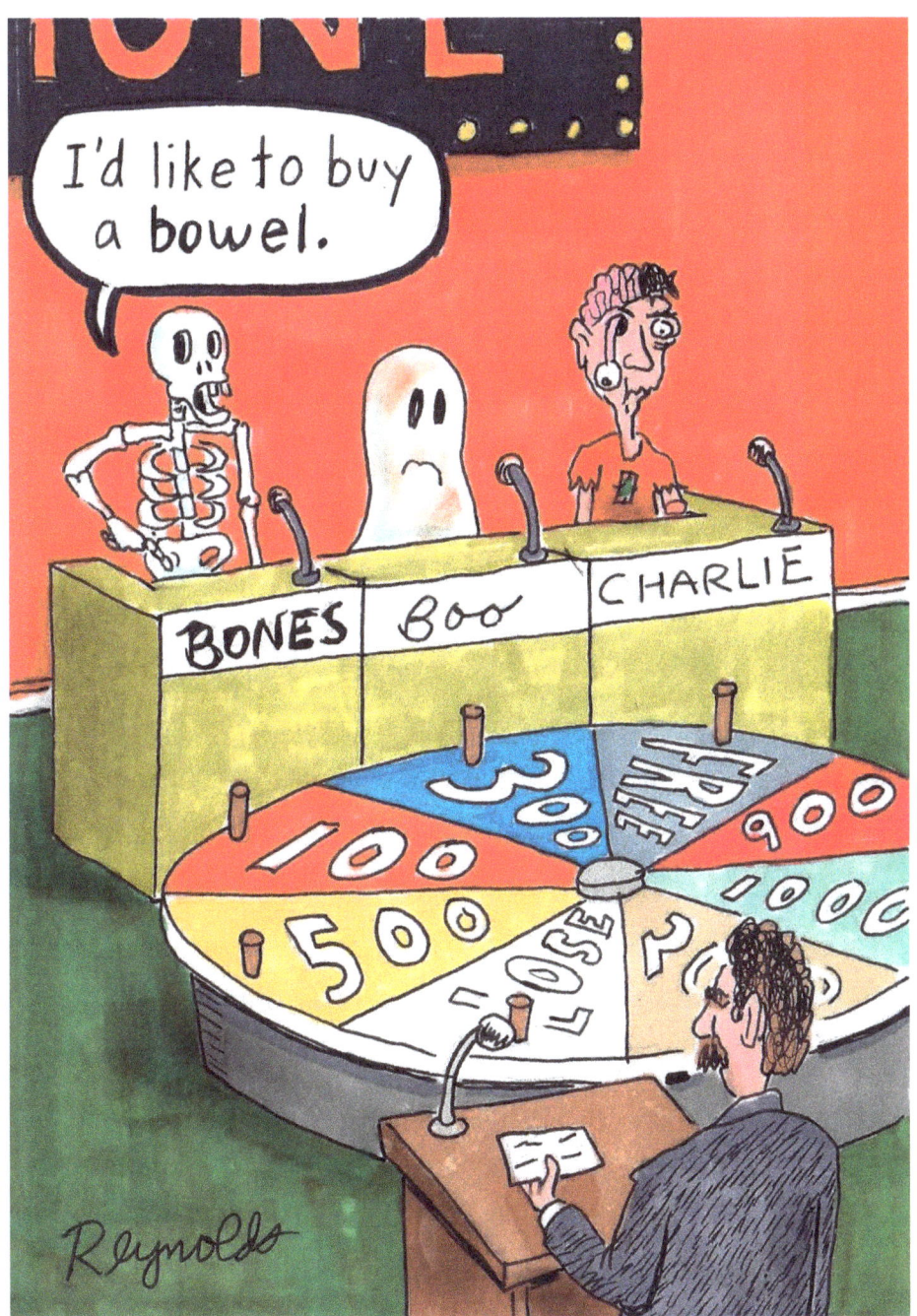

There are over one thousand six hundred known digestive enzymes.

Drinking a cold carbonated beverage will release more gas than drinking a warm carbonated beverage. This is based on the physical principle of Charles's Law, which describes how temperature changes affect pressure.

A glass filled to the brim can have a level of fluid above the edge of the glass that does not overflow. This is because of the physical property of surface tension of the fluid.

Without stomach acid digestion can still take place, but at a slower pace.

The air we inhale contains less than one tenth of one percent carbon dioxide, the air we exhale has levels of carbon dioxide that is typically one hundred times as great.

The Fart Side: Windbreaks!

"The good news is that you don't have mad cow's disease. The bad news is you're lactose intolerant."

Spices, especially ginger and curcumin, stimulate the liver to secrete more bile, and the pancreas to secrete more lipase, both if which help you digest fat.

Pouring the invisible gas carbon dioxide into a glass container holding a lit candle at its bottom will cause the flame to be extinguished. This is because the heavier than air carbon dioxide will displace the air at the bottom that contains the oxygen the flame requires.

The primary physiologic stimulus for breathing is the level of carbon dioxide in the blood, not the level of oxygen that many incorrectly believe is responsible.

Reflux is common during pregnancy due to both the growing baby in the uterus, as well as the high levels of the hormone progesterone which relaxes the lower esophageal sphincter.

The Fart Side: Windbreaks!

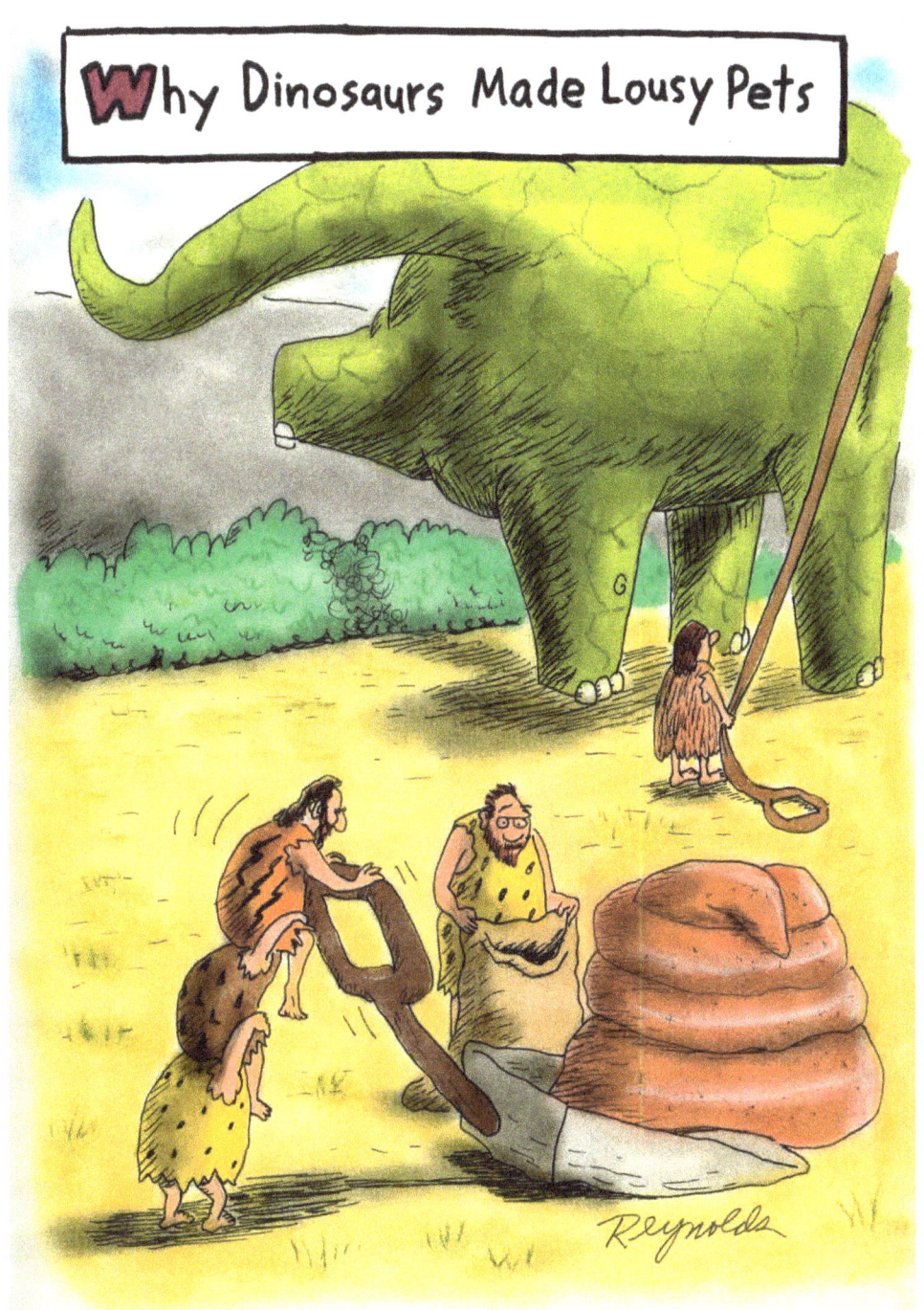

Humans who overeat carrots develop skin carrot color pigmentation because of carotenemia, excessive carotenoids in the blood.

The air hunger of near suffocation is derived from excess carbon dioxide buildup, not lack of oxygen. It is for this reason that breathing helium for the humor of a squeaky Donald Duck voice is very dangerous. As long as the carbon dioxide is being exhaled, the victim is not aware that they are being deprived of oxygen until death occurs suddenly.

A chocolate, mint, or other herbal carminative are often offered on leaving a restaurant to relax the lower esophageal sphincter. This is done to allow air swallowed during a meal to be released by burping, making the diner more comfortable. Notice how it is offered as you leave the restaurant, so that you do not burp on their premises.

The Fart Side: Windbreaks!

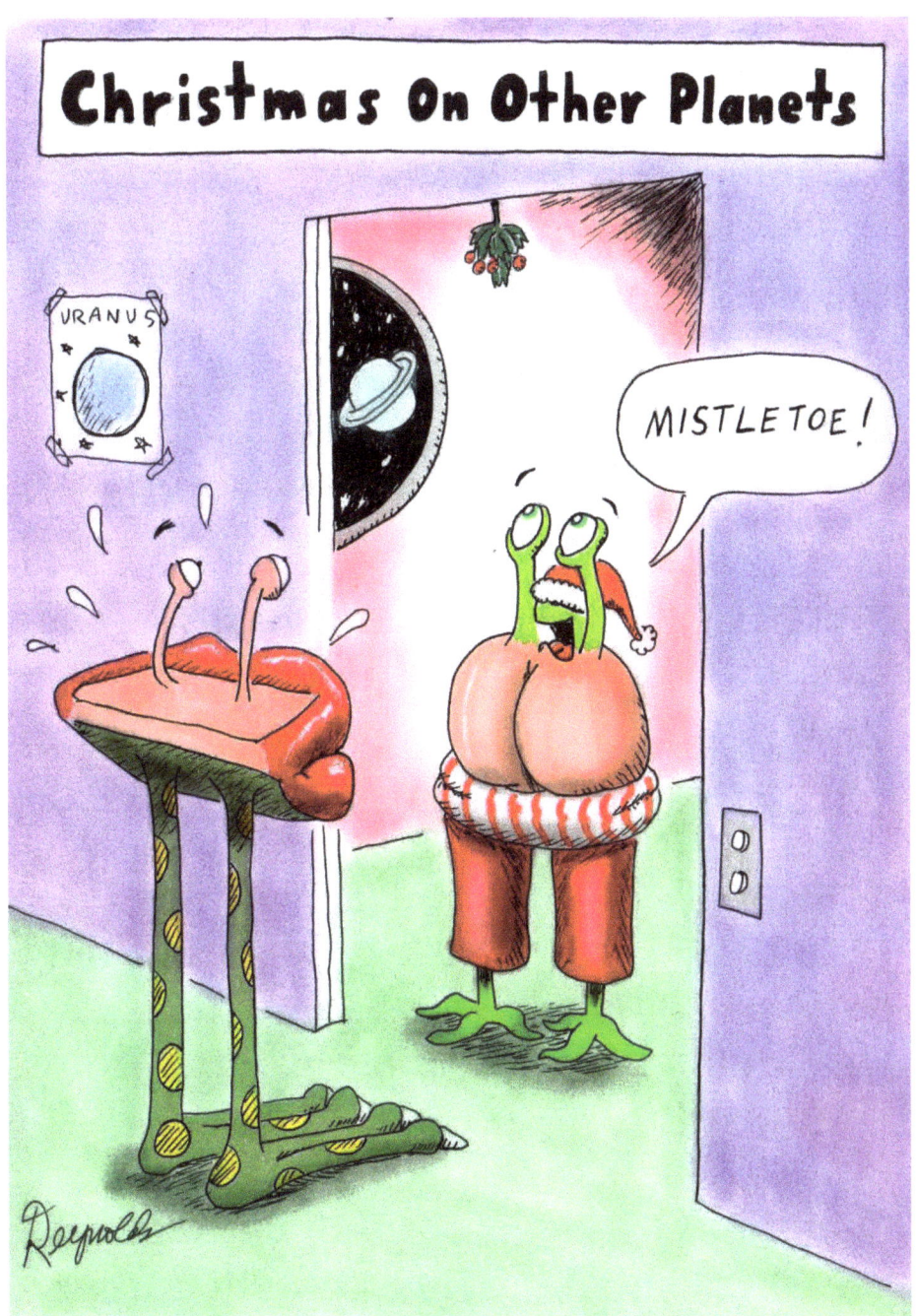

Governments have considered instituting taxes on livestock because of their global warming contribution. They belch and fart enormous quantities of methane into the atmosphere.

Lighting a cow manure patty is an unsafe way to demonstrate that they are flammable.

Although it is not recommended, you can swallow while standing on your head. The strength of peristalsis can overcome the force of gravity.

Drowning victims frequently float to the surface hours to days after being at the bottom of a pool of water, because of the continuation of intestinal gas formation after death.

Flamingoes are usually pink because they eat lots of shrimp, which contain the color pigment carotenoids in their bodies.

The Fart Side: Windbreaks!

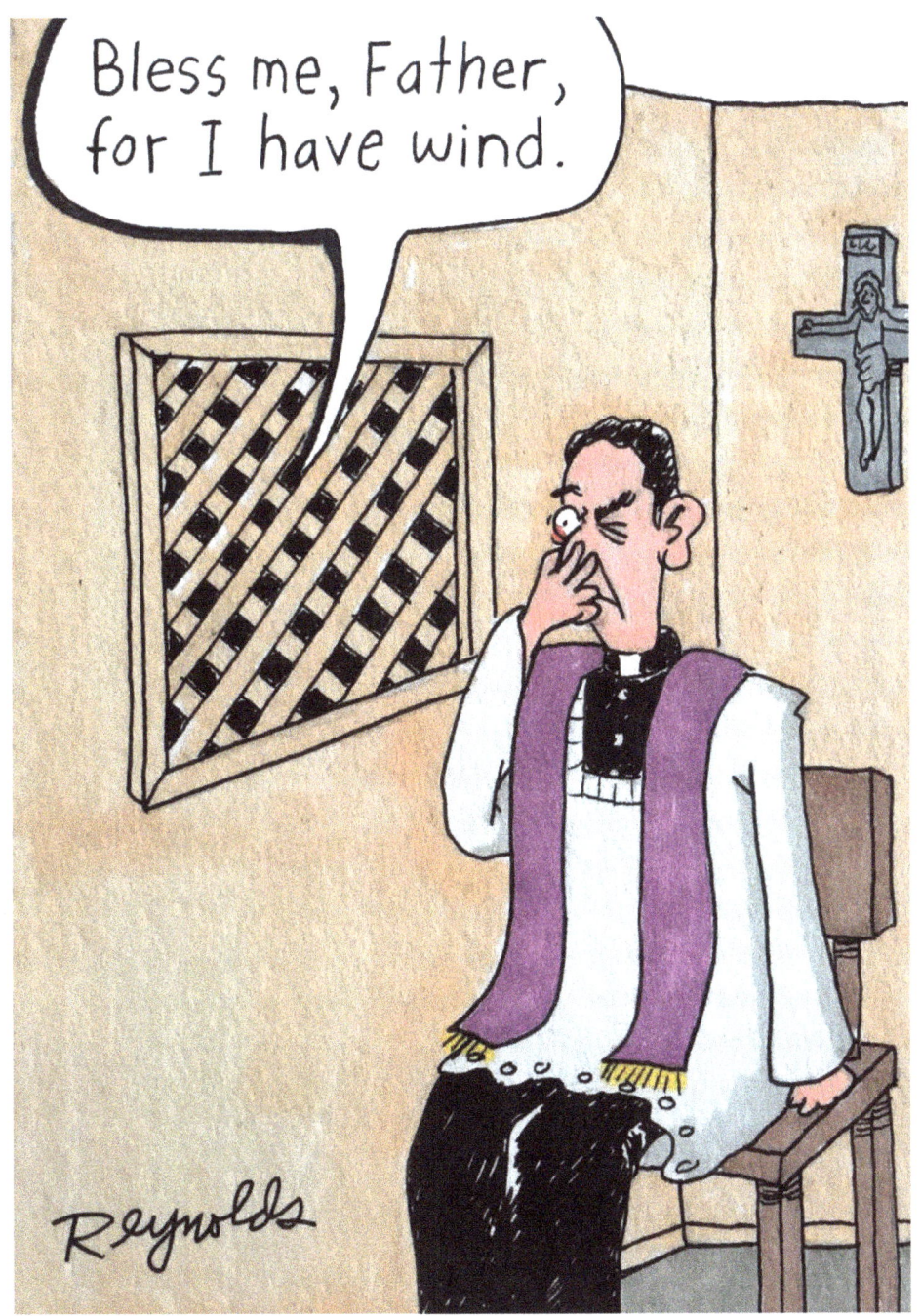

Jaundice can be distinguished from carotenemia because jaundice will discolor the whites (sclera) of the eyes yellow, while in carotenemia the sclera remains white.

Pumpernickel is the German word for 'Devil's Farts' and the coarse grain of the bread leads to farting.

Raw Lima beans contain cyanide and can cause illness and death if consumed in excess.

Swallowing of a liquid is more complex and challenging than the swallowing of a solid.

Eating and chewing raw castor beans can be fatal because of the ricin toxin.

The pastry delicacy Pets de Nonne ('Nun's Farts' in French) are so named because they are heavenly light and airy.

The Fart Side: Windbreaks!

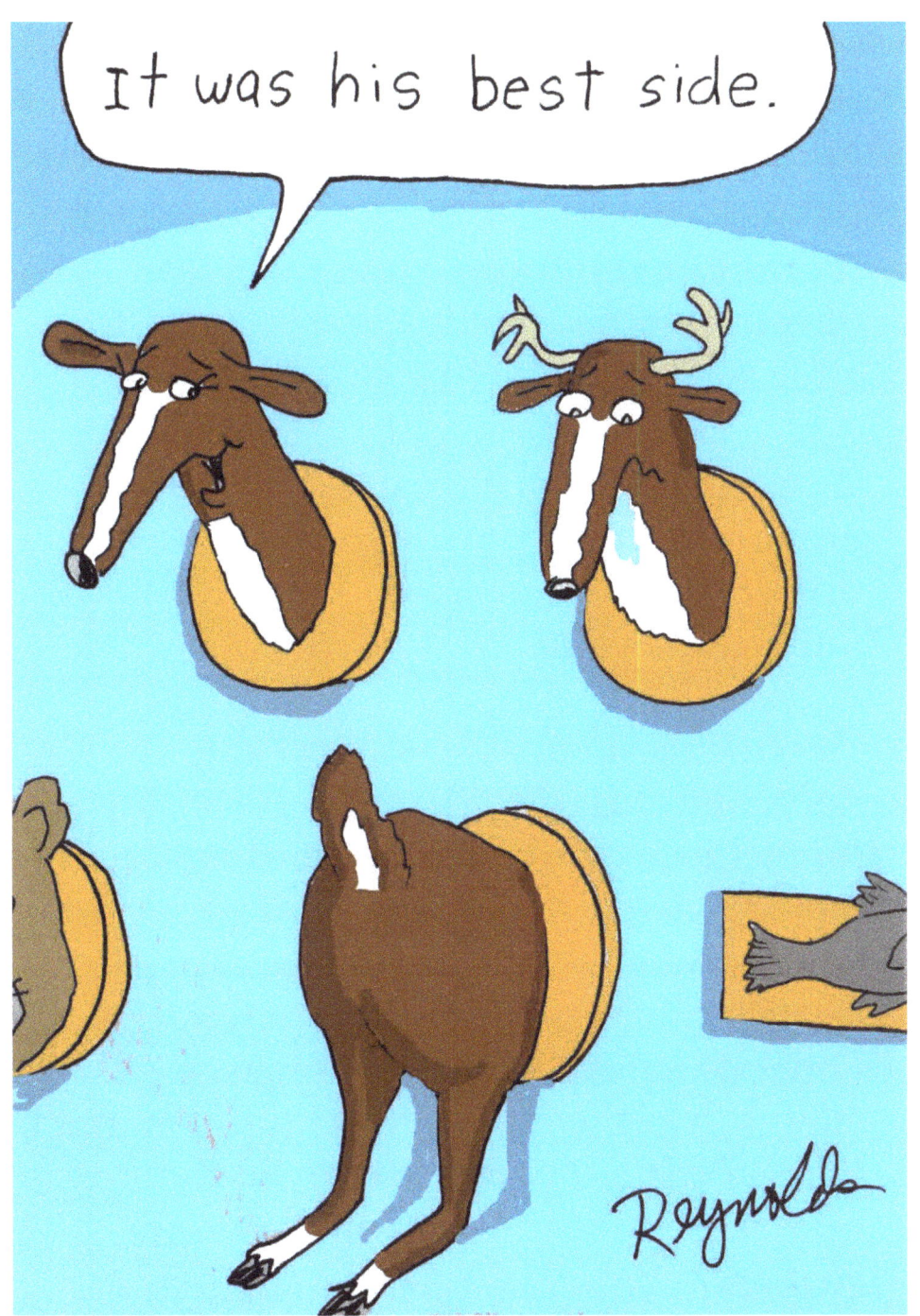

In the mouth, food is either cooled or warmed to a more suitable temperature for the internal organs.

It is not uncommon to temporarily develop lactose (milk sugar) intolerance after a gastroenteritis with diarrhea.

Human digestion does not remove all nutrient value from the food ingested, so the waste product of feces has remaining nutritional value.

Morticians secure the anus of the deceased closed so that an audible fart form the corpse or casket does not frighten attendees at a memorial service or funeral.

Coprophagia, the eating of feces, is common in the animal world, and is much more frequent inadvertently in the human population than most people realize.

The Fart Side: Windbreaks!

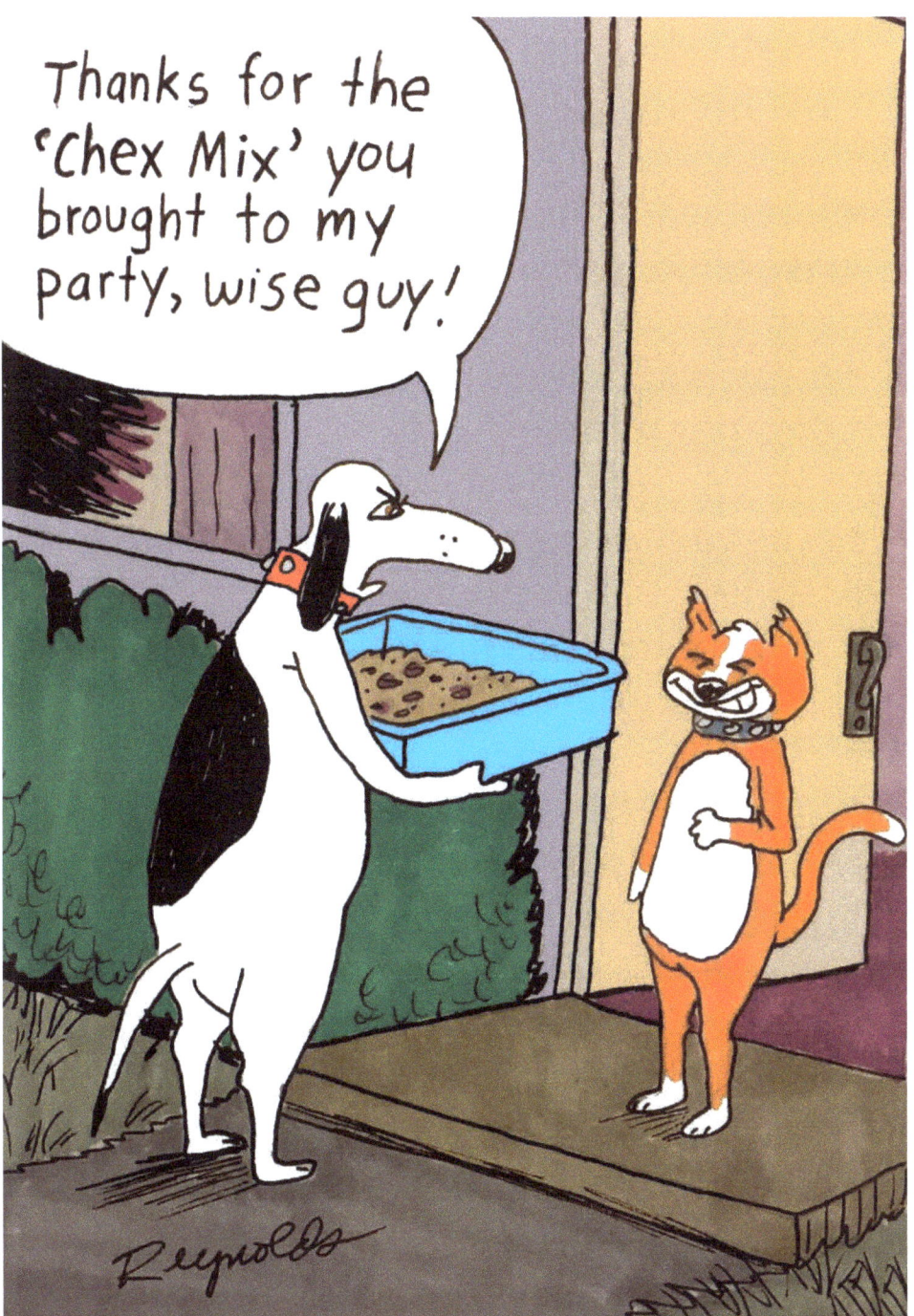

Dough rises with the yeast producing carbon dioxide gas by fermentation.

The characteristic holes in Swiss cheese arise from microbial gas production.

The average speed of a cough is thirty miles per hour.

Feces harboring a virus that causes diarrhea may contain more than ten trillion infectious particles in one gram (less than one-thirtieth of an ounce).

Budweiser beer broadcast a humorous Super Bowl advertisement viewed by millions featuring a flammable horse fart.

Regular dental flossing decreases the risk of cardiovascular disease.

Pineapple contains the protease enzyme bromelain, which breaks down protein and can be used as a meat tenderizer.

The Fart Side: Windbreaks!

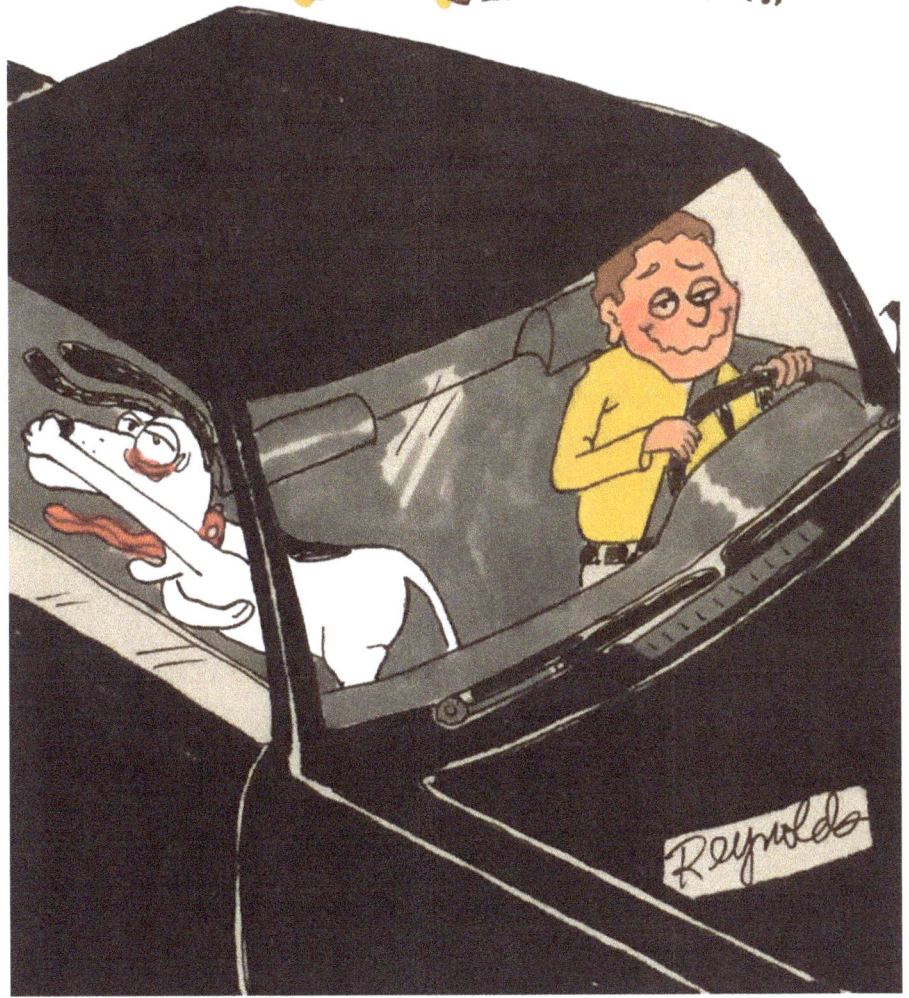

Farting has become more accepted in Western society, with products to address it advertised openly.

The average speed velocity of a sneeze is ninety-five miles per hour.

Fecal microbiota transplantation has become the treatment of choice for several medical conditions.

Papaya contains the protease enzyme papain, which breaks down protein and can be used as a meat tenderizer.

Unfortunately, neither science nor the Guinness Book of Records offers information on the average speed of a fart, but the diffusion of its smell has been recorded as greater than ten miles per hour.

Internal bleeding, iron, bismuth, and black liquorice cause black stool.

The Fart Side: Windbreaks!

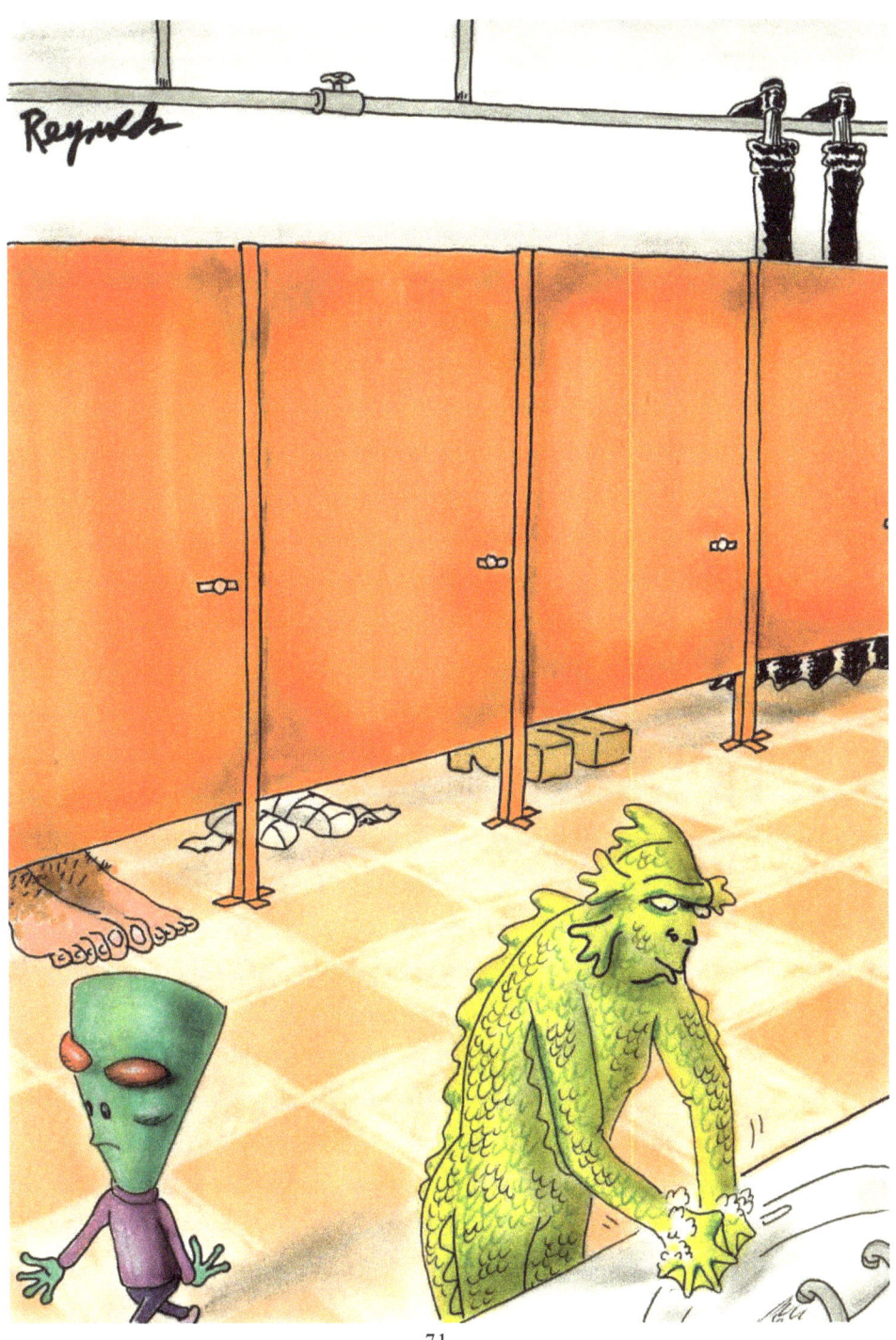

Chewing food breaks it down into smaller pieces, aiding digestion and accelerating passage through the stomach, which would otherwise have to work harder.

Although dietary fiber cannot be digested by humans, it is an important part of the diet serving as a prebiotic to keep the gut microbiome healthy.

The colon is not a vital organ, and people can live a normal life span without it.

Some individuals have gut microbes that ferment sugars into alcohol that is subsequently absorbed. It can lead to intoxication without ever having had a drink of alcohol.

Hydrogen is a flammable gas, and is the most abundant element in the universe. It comprises ninety-eight percent of the mass of known matter. Another one percent of the total mass is helium.

The Fart Side: Windbreaks!

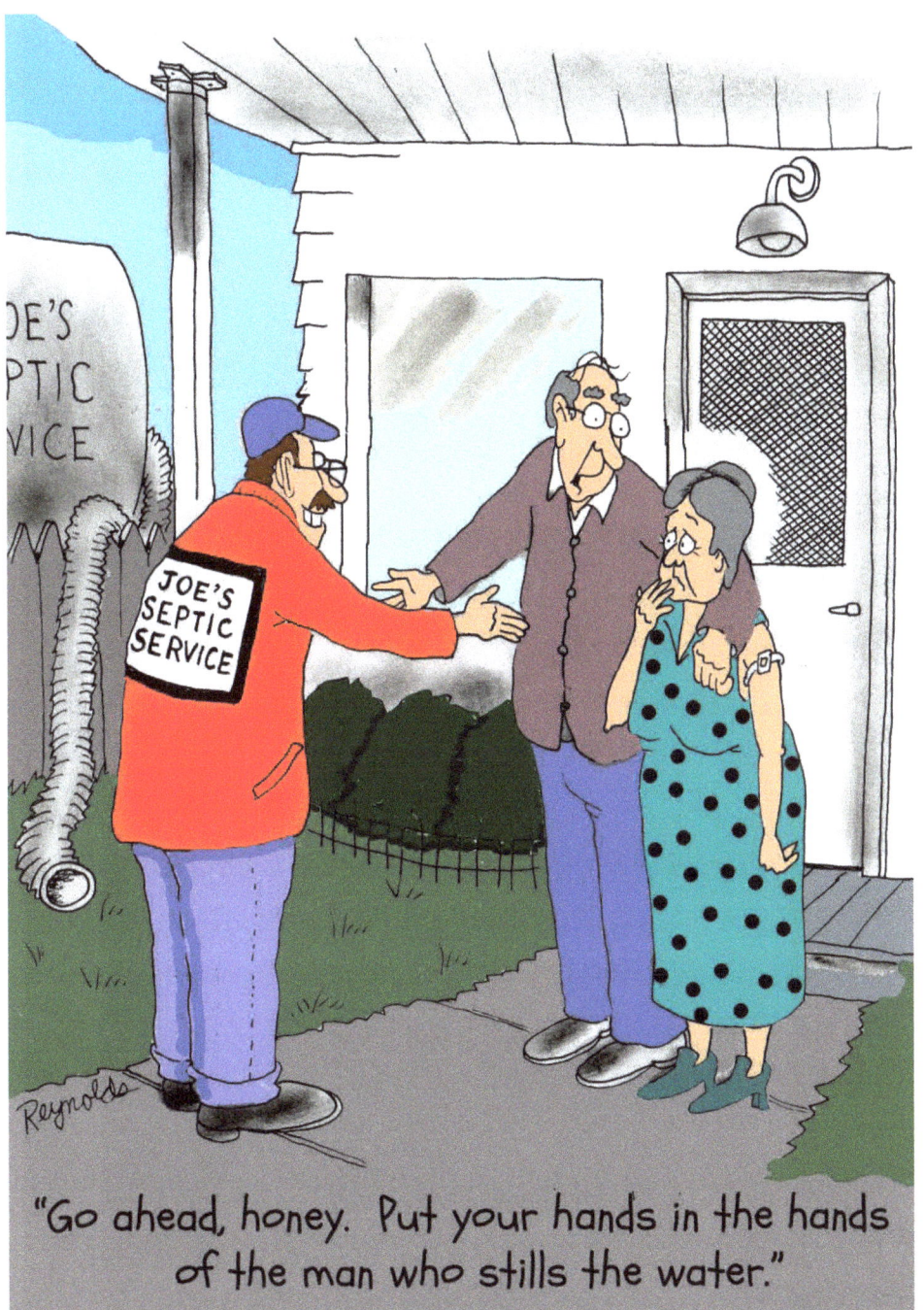

Mechanical grinding of chewing disrupts the cell walls of plants, aiding in human digestion by allowing enzymes to access the cell content.

The field of study of the gut brain, also known as the enteric nervous system, is called neurogastroenterology.

Petroleum and oil deposits originated from decomposing organic material. They became liquefied over millions of years under enormous pressure thousands of feet underground.

One milliliter (one-fifth of a teaspoon) of seawater can harbor over two hundred and fifty million viral bacteriophages. This is an important part of the microbiome.

Viral bacteriophages kill bacteria and can be more effective than antibiotics in the treatment of certain infections.

The Fart Side: Windbreaks!

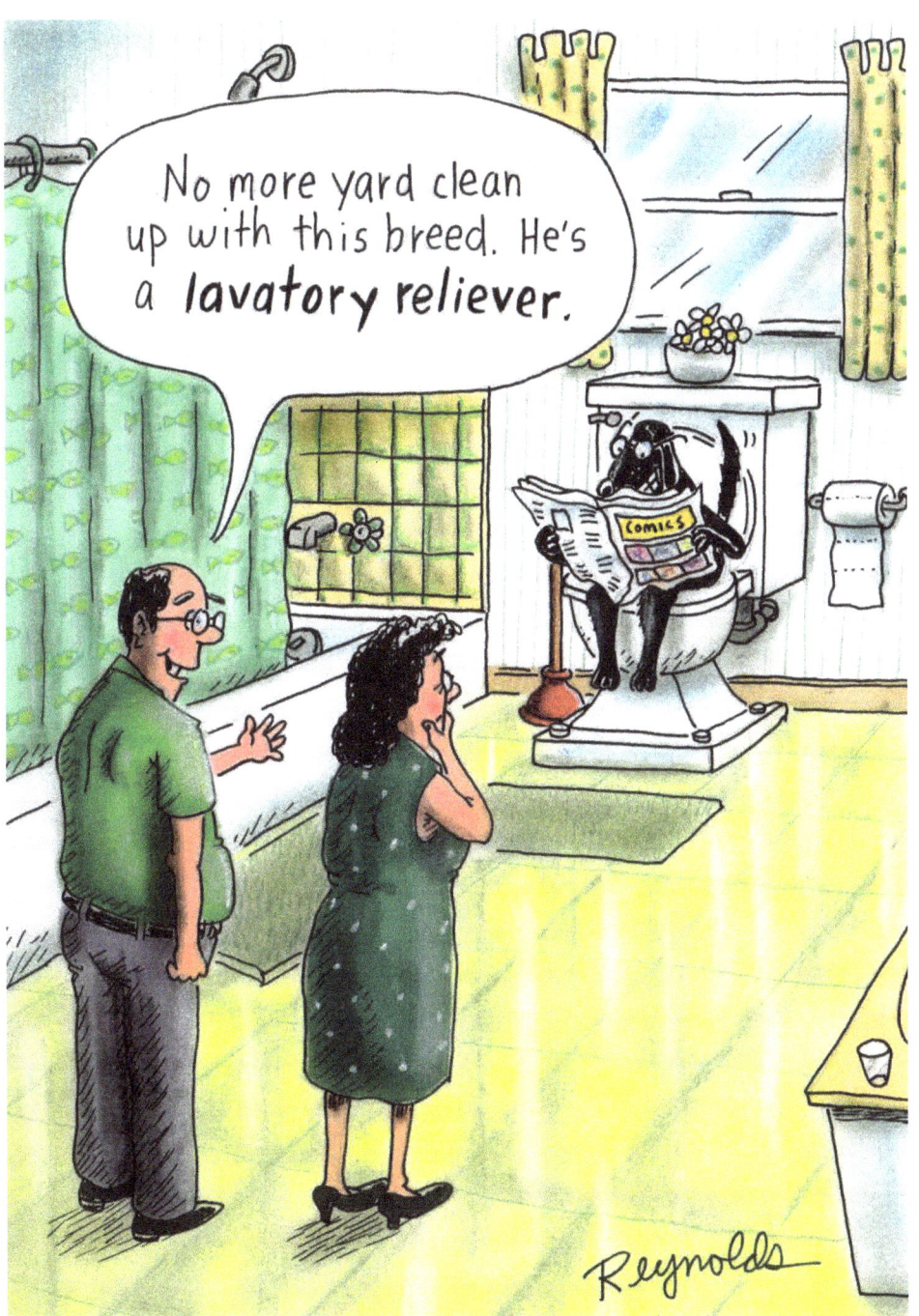

The average cow produces manure that release enough methane to power a one-hundred-watt light bulb for twenty-four hours.

The most common source of methane, comprising over twenty-five percent of the amount found in the atmosphere, is from termite farts. The microbes in the termite's guts generate the methane from the cellulose the termites ingest as their diet.

Some microbes reproduce so quickly that their population can double every twenty minutes. With exponential growth rates, they can quickly overwhelm the victim, and lead to a rapid fatal infection.

Over fifty percent of the biomass on Earth are comprised of bacteria and Archaea. Their population number is estimated to be five quintillion (five followed by thirty zeroes).

The Fart Side: Windbreaks!

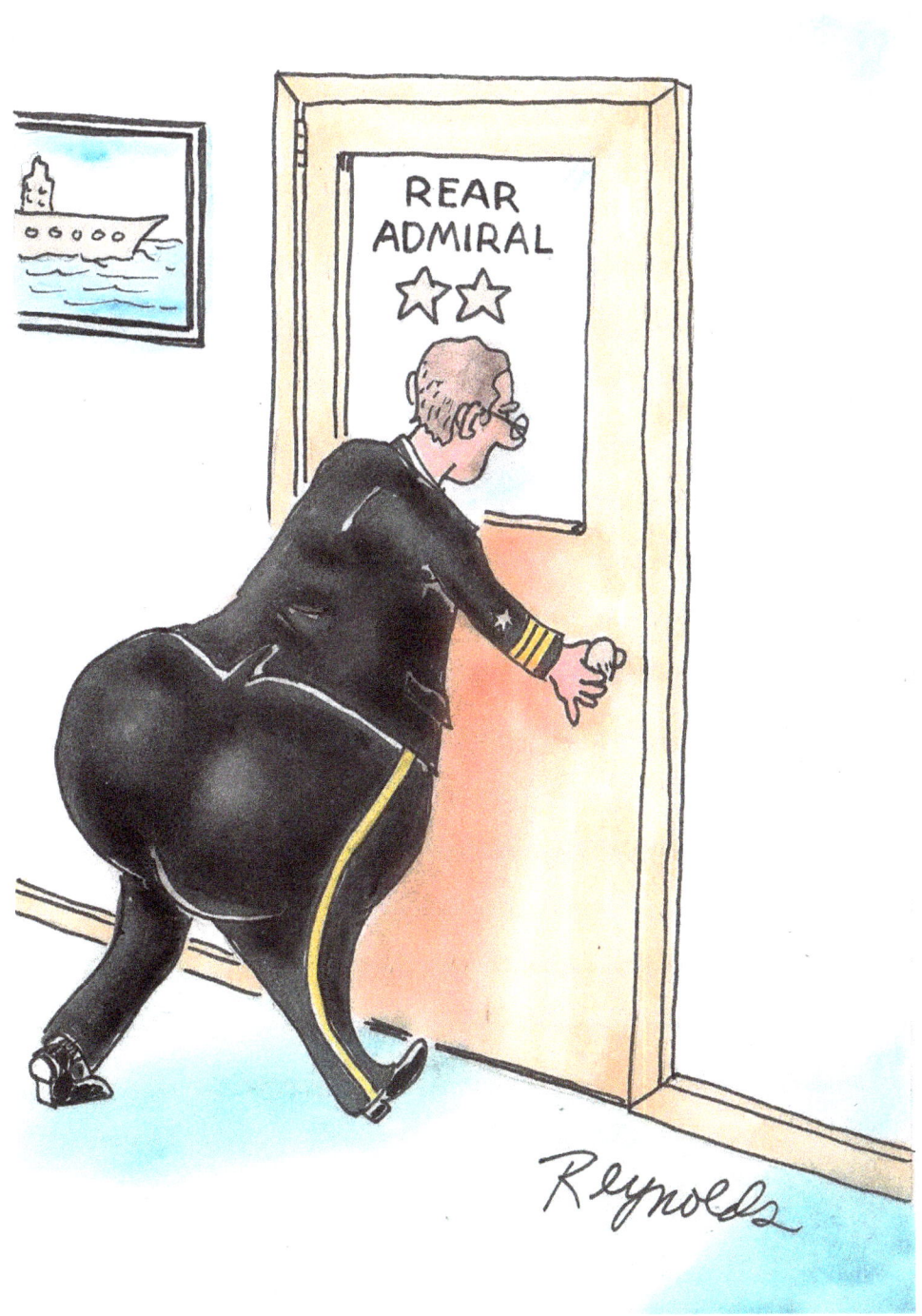

Although oxygen is vital to human life, it's high reactivity leads to cellular damage, inflammation, aging, and death.

Over seventy percent of the free oxygen in the earth's atmosphere is generated by marine Cyanobacteria and green algae.

Human blood turns bright red when the iron rich hemoglobin binds to oxygen.

The blood of mollusks and crabs turns bright blue when the copper rich hemocyanin binds to oxygen.

Many people who suffer from GERD (GastroEsophageal Reflux Disease) do not have heartburn. Other signs and symptoms may include asthma, cough, sinus conditions, sore throat, laryngitis, dental caries (cavities), loss of tooth enamel, hoarseness, hiccups, pneumonia, bronchitis, and other conditions.

The Fart Side: Windbreaks!

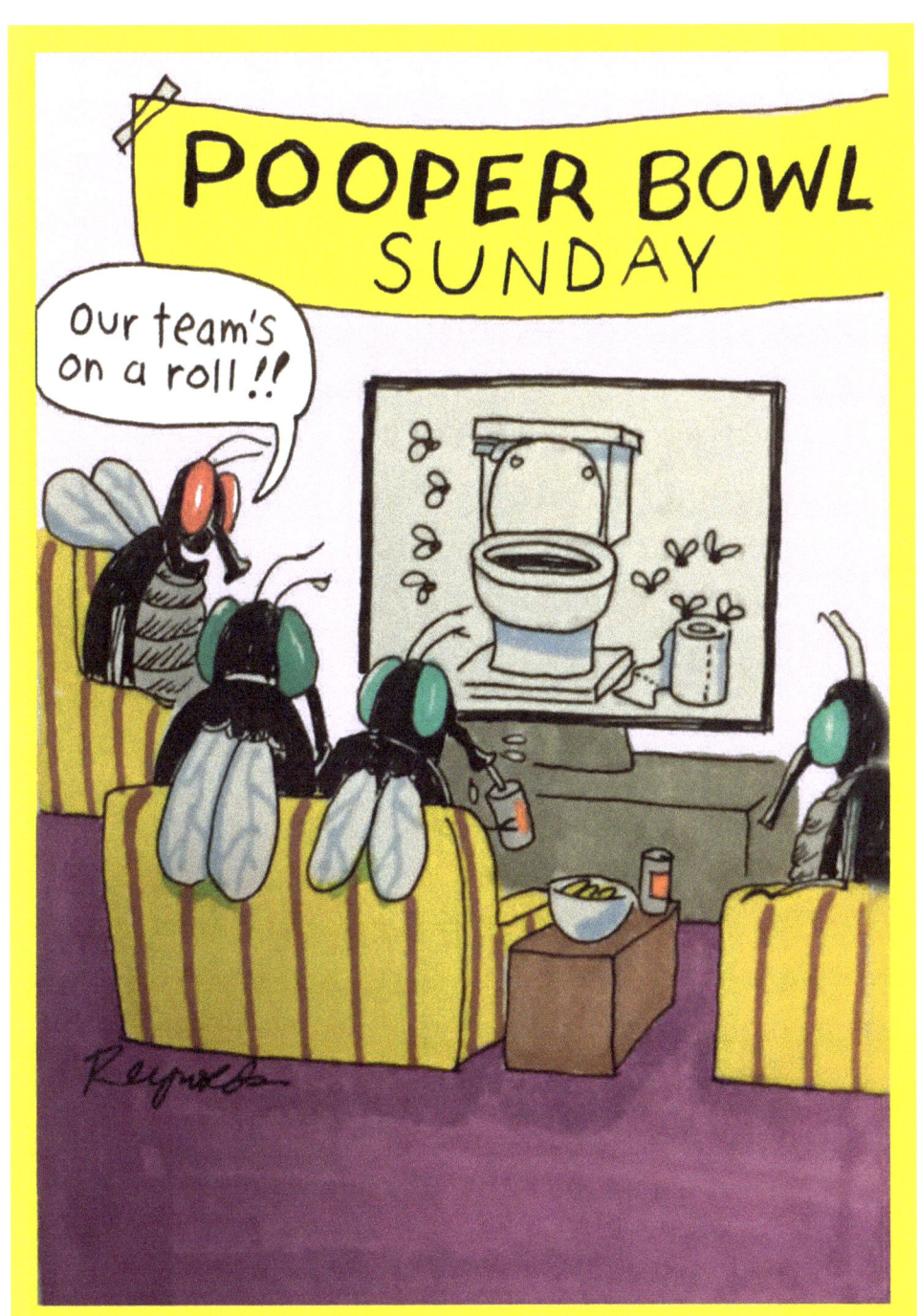

An iron nail will gain weight as it rusts. This is because it incorporates oxygen as it oxidizes while rusting.

There was a time in Earth history, about three hundred million years ago, when the oxygen level in the atmosphere was thirty-five percent. This is very high compared to today's level of about twenty-one percent. Fossil records from that time period show that insect wingspans were often over two feet wide.

Billions of humans are infested and infected with parasites.

In the US over twenty percent of the adult population has been infected with the Toxoplasma parasite harbored by cats. It is very dangerous to the fetus during human pregnancy.

William Shakespeare refers to a fart in one of his plays.

The Fart Side: Windbreaks!

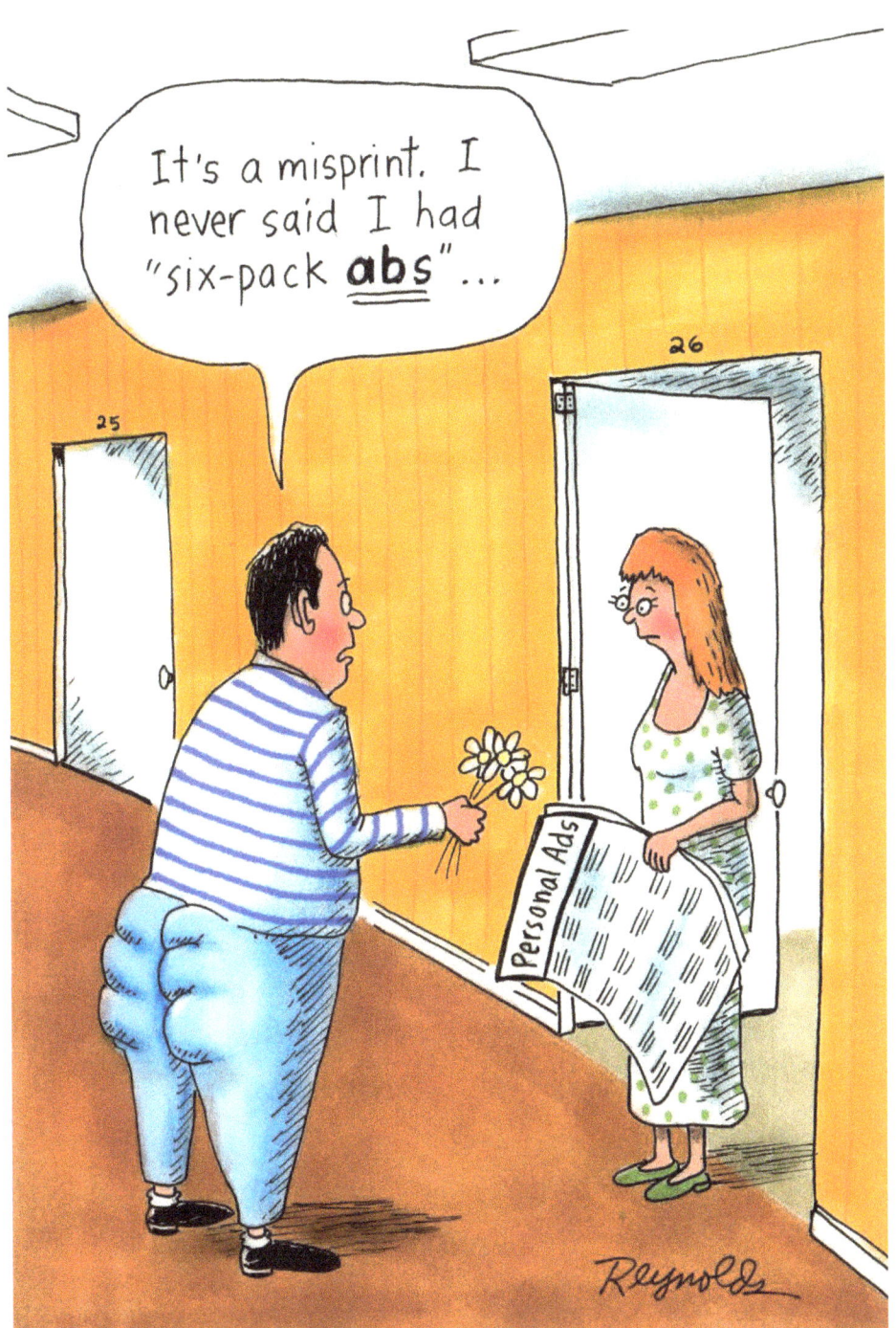

Many experts suggest at least forty chews per bite of food. The extra chewing aids digestion, burns calories in the process, and reduces food intake.

American statesman Benjamin Franklin wrote an essay on farts as a practical joke on a scientific society.

US President Lyndon Johnson insulted future US President Gerald Ford by claiming he wasn't smart enough to be able to chew gum and fart at the same time.

Roman Emperor Claudius decreed that citizens of Rome were allowed to fart in public, because he believed that holding back a fart could lead to illness or death.

The famous composer Richard Wagner often complained about his bowel problems, and described his farts by the musical notes and keys they played.

The Fart Side: Windbreaks!

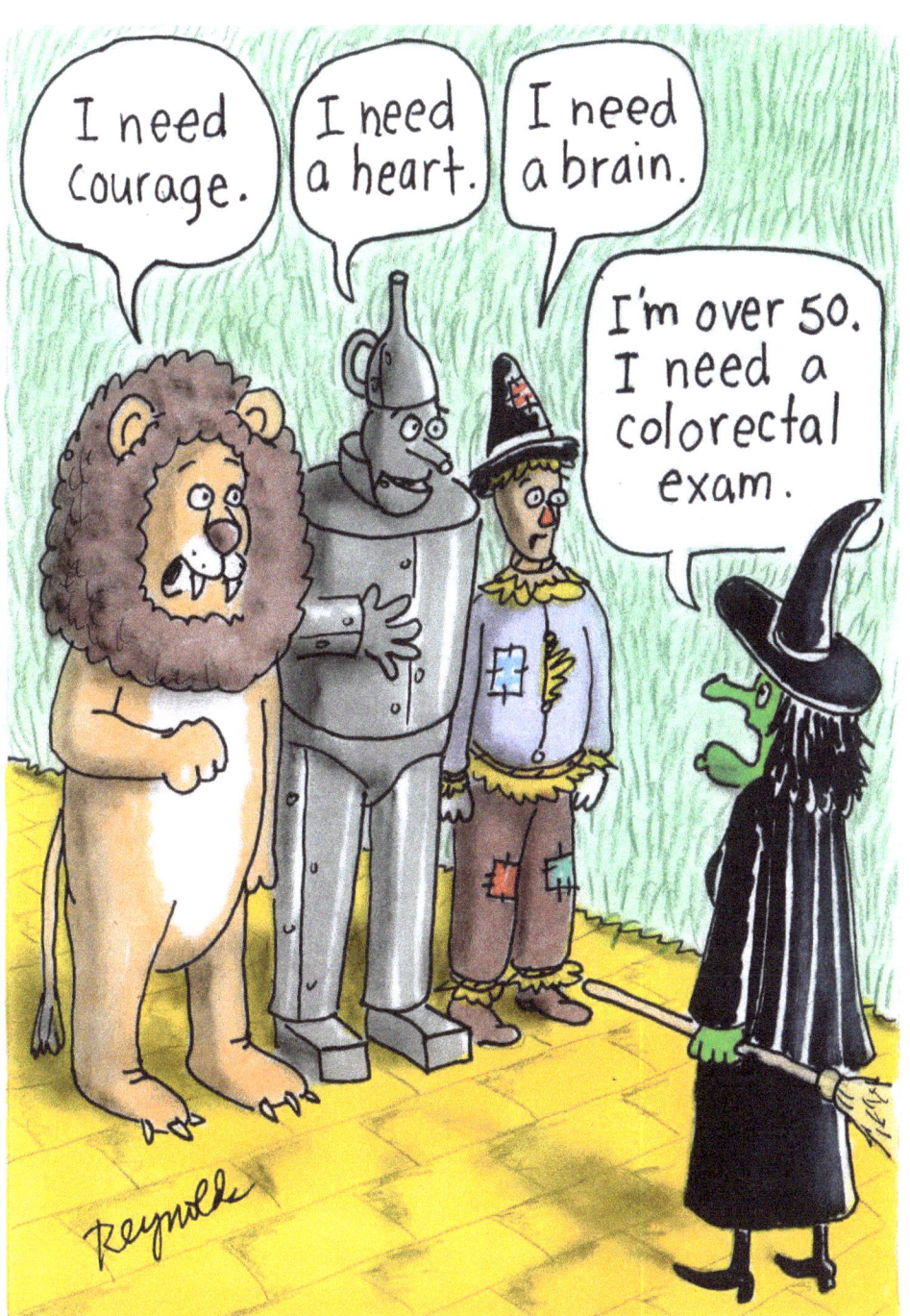

Without chewing breaking down the plant cell walls made of cellulose, humans would not be able to digest plants since we do not have the enzyme cellulase.

Wolfgang Amadeus Mozart was fascinated and obsessed with farts and scatological matter.

Joseph Pujol, known by the name Le Pétomane (The Farter Maniac in French) was the highest paid stage performer of his day. He played Le Marseilles and other tunes by farting them out of his human wind instrument, his butt, on the Moulin Rouge in Paris.

Prominent fart scenes have occurred in over one hundred Hollywood movies, including Walt Disney films for children.

Toilet flush handles have four hundred times as many bacterial contaminants as the toilet seat.

The Fart Side: Windbreaks!

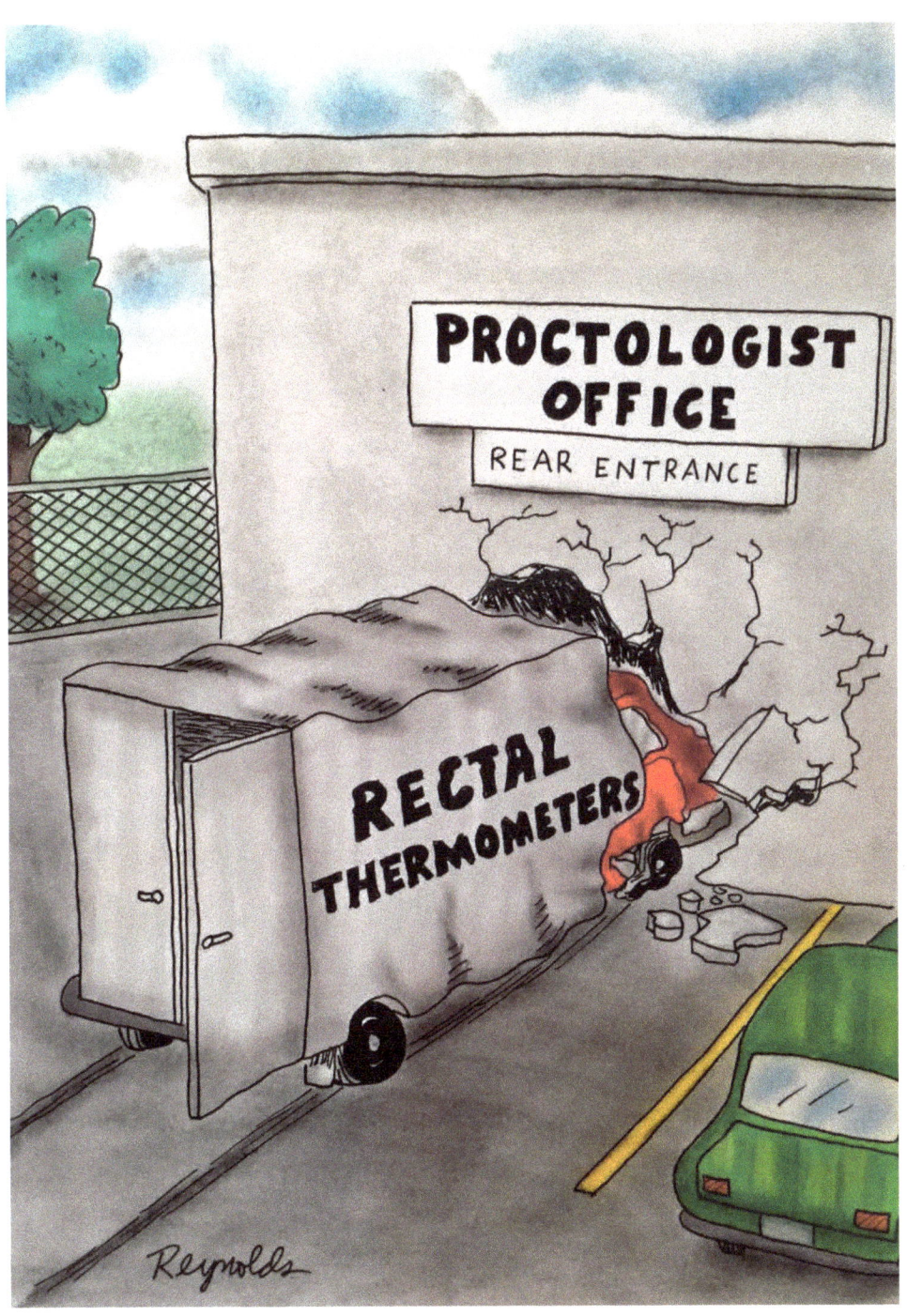

There are over one hundred million nerve cells in the enteric nervous system. That's more neurons than are found in the spinal cord or peripheral nervous system.

Animal dung is a major fuel source in some parts of the world.

The caloric energy found in food is only partially absorbed with digestion.

Ruminant livestock such as cattle generate more methane from burping than farting.

Gelato compared to ice cream has a lower calorie content by weight, but a higher calorie content by volume.

The potency and aroma of the farts of boys increases as they go through puberty and reach adulthood. Eating meat will contribute to the aroma.

The Fart Side: Windbreaks!

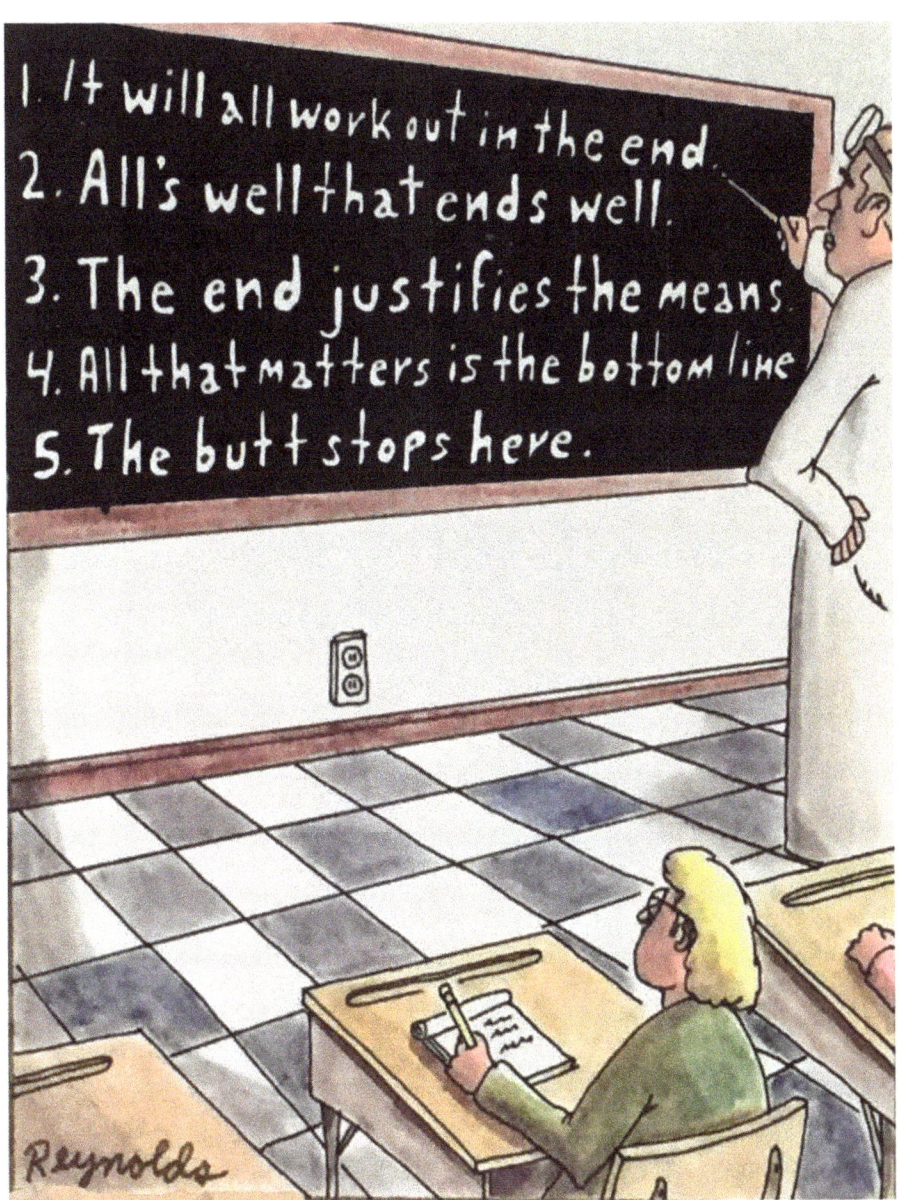

Philosophy Class For Proctology Students

Up to ninety percent of the fibers of the vagus nerve carry information from the gut to the brain, rather than the other way around.

Alcoholic beverages, typically containing 1% to 40% ethanol by volume, have been produced and consumed by humans since pre-historic times.

The saliva secreted in the resting mouth is not identical to the saliva when eating.

Females have a heightened sense of smell at the time of ovulation during the menstrual cycle.

Normal stomach acid can dissolve a metallic object in minutes.

Enzymes can be effective for multiple reactions with the substrate, and act as a catalyst. They remain unchanged, retaining activity after the reaction.

The Fart Side: Windbreaks!

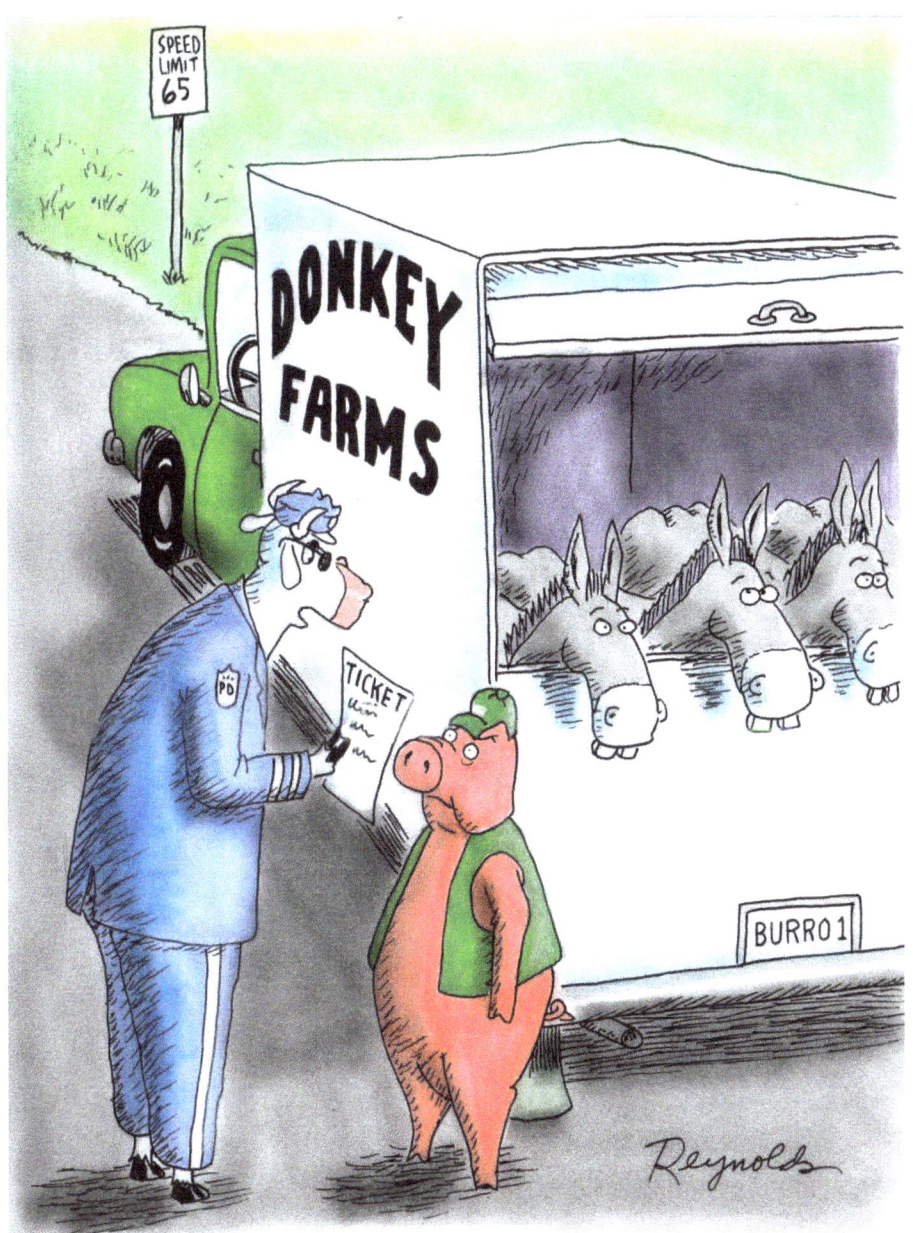

"It's not for speeding. It's for hauling ass."

Over ninety percent of the serotonin in the human body, one of the major neurotransmitters, is found in the gut.

Most seeds generate and release the specific active enzyme needed to digest the plant starch present with germination.

In Japan, the fecal waste of rich people was more expensive as a fertilizer, known as night soil. It was thought to have greater nutritional value because of their better diet.

Methane is twenty times as potent a greenhouse gas as carbon dioxide.

Injury and death can occur because of intestinal gas leading to barotrauma after excessive expansion. This occurs when going from higher to lower atmospheric pressure, such as going from below sea level to high altitude.

The Fart Side: Windbreaks!

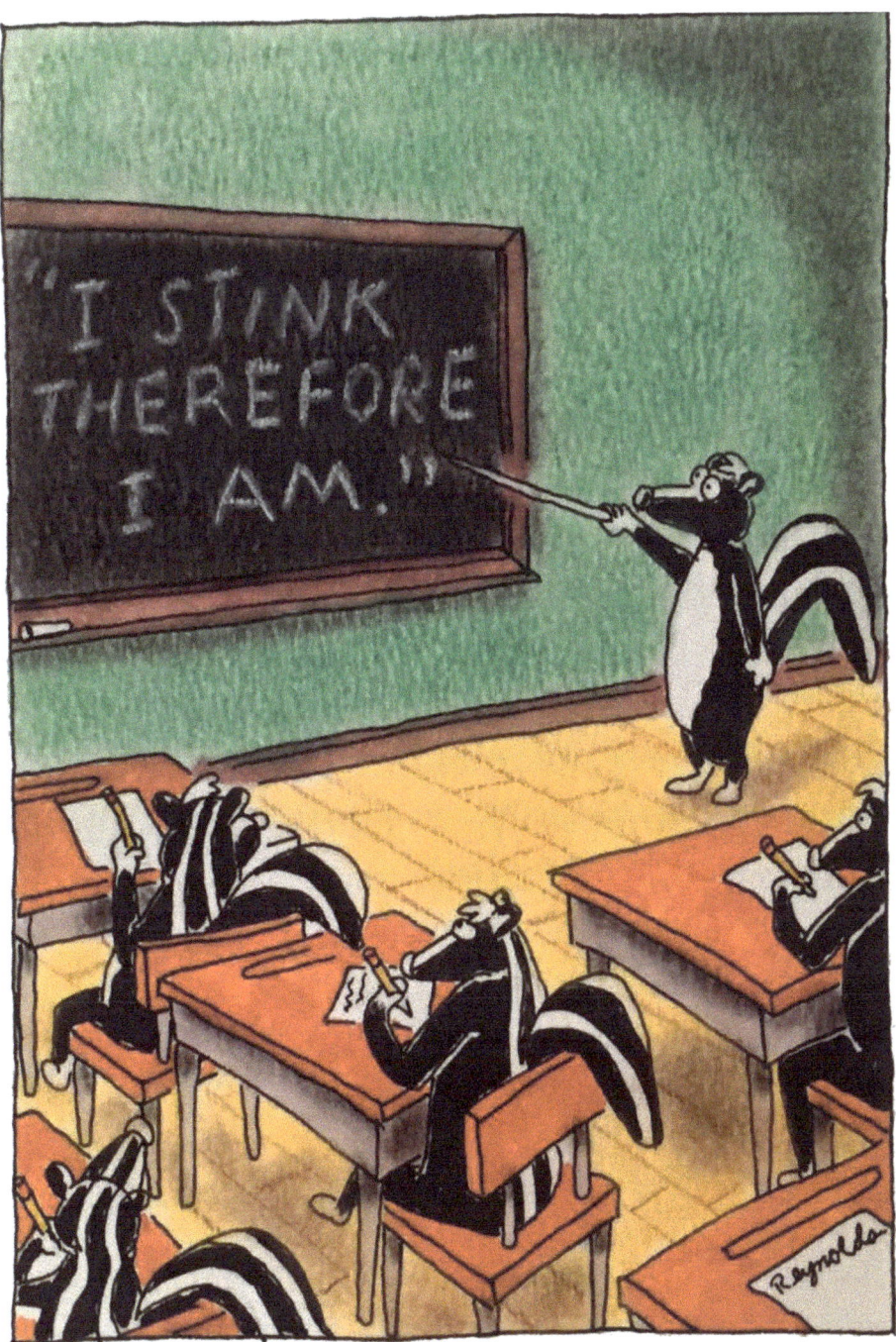

Texture of food and 'mouthfeel' is transmitted via the Trigeminal Cranial Nerve

The intestines of a horse are eighty-nine feet long.

Popular antidepressants, known as SSRI's (Selective Serotonin Reuptake Inhibitors, e.g. Prozac, Paxil) work by elevating the body level of serotonin.

Carbon Dioxide gas is easily absorbed by the gut, enters into solution in the blood, and is eliminated from the body by being exhaled via the lungs

Seventy-five percent of African-American, Jewish, Native American, and Mexican American populations are lactose intolerant.

A specialist seller of cheese is sometimes known as a cheese monger.

The Fart Side: Windbreaks!

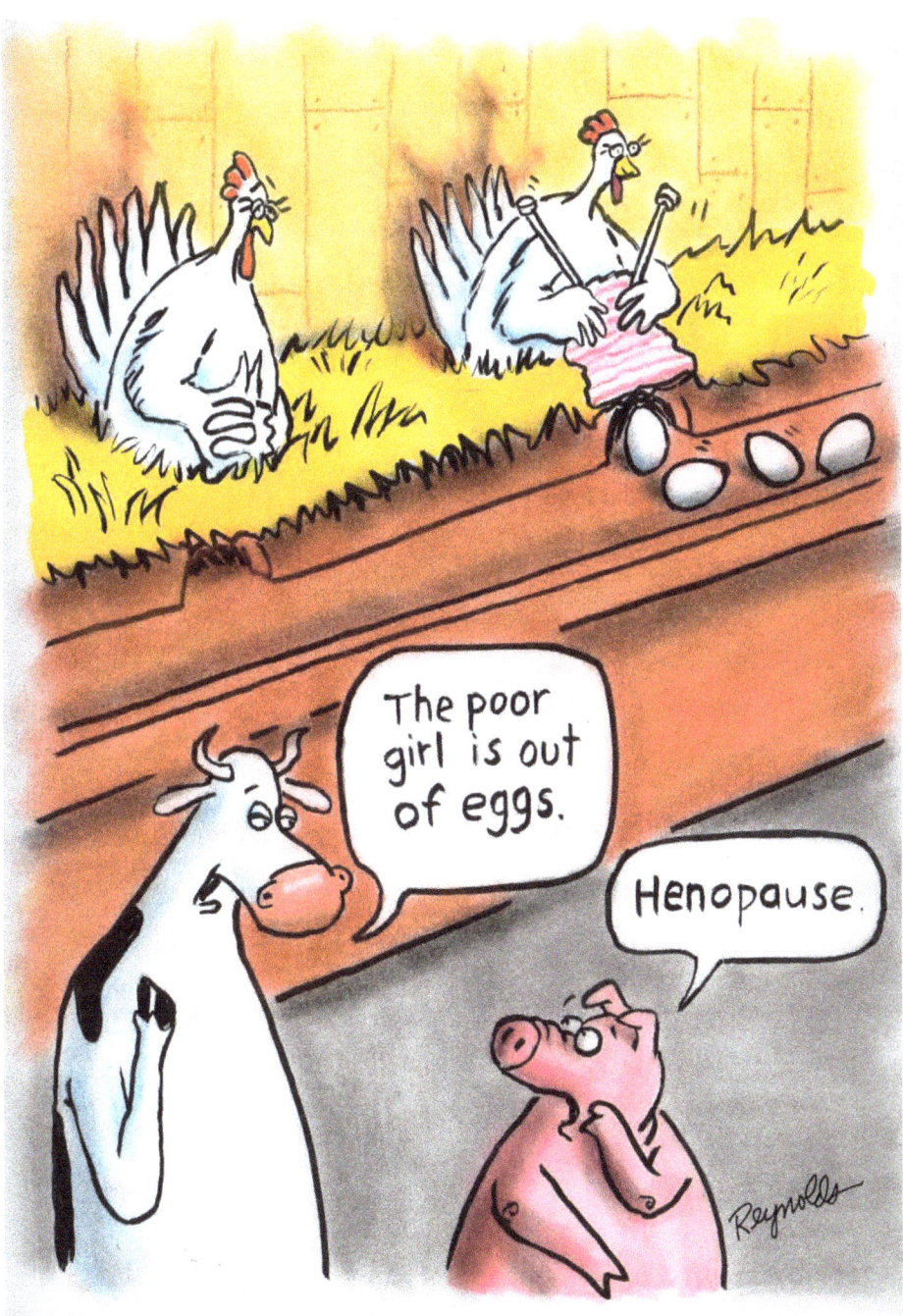

Breathing helium to make your voice sound like Donald Duck is not a safe way to have fun. The risk of asphyxiation is increased. The respiratory reflex is not triggered by lack of oxygen alone.

Heartburn is common in pregnancy, partly because of the high levels of the hormone progesterone, which relaxes the lower esophageal sphincter.

Farting is more likely to occur in elevators while they are going up in high rise buildings than in those exact same elevators going down because of the change in atmospheric pressure.

Animal dung is a major fuel source in some parts of the world. The caloric energy found in food is only partially absorbed with digestion.

Ruminant livestock such as cattle generate most methane from burping.

The Fart Side: Windbreaks!

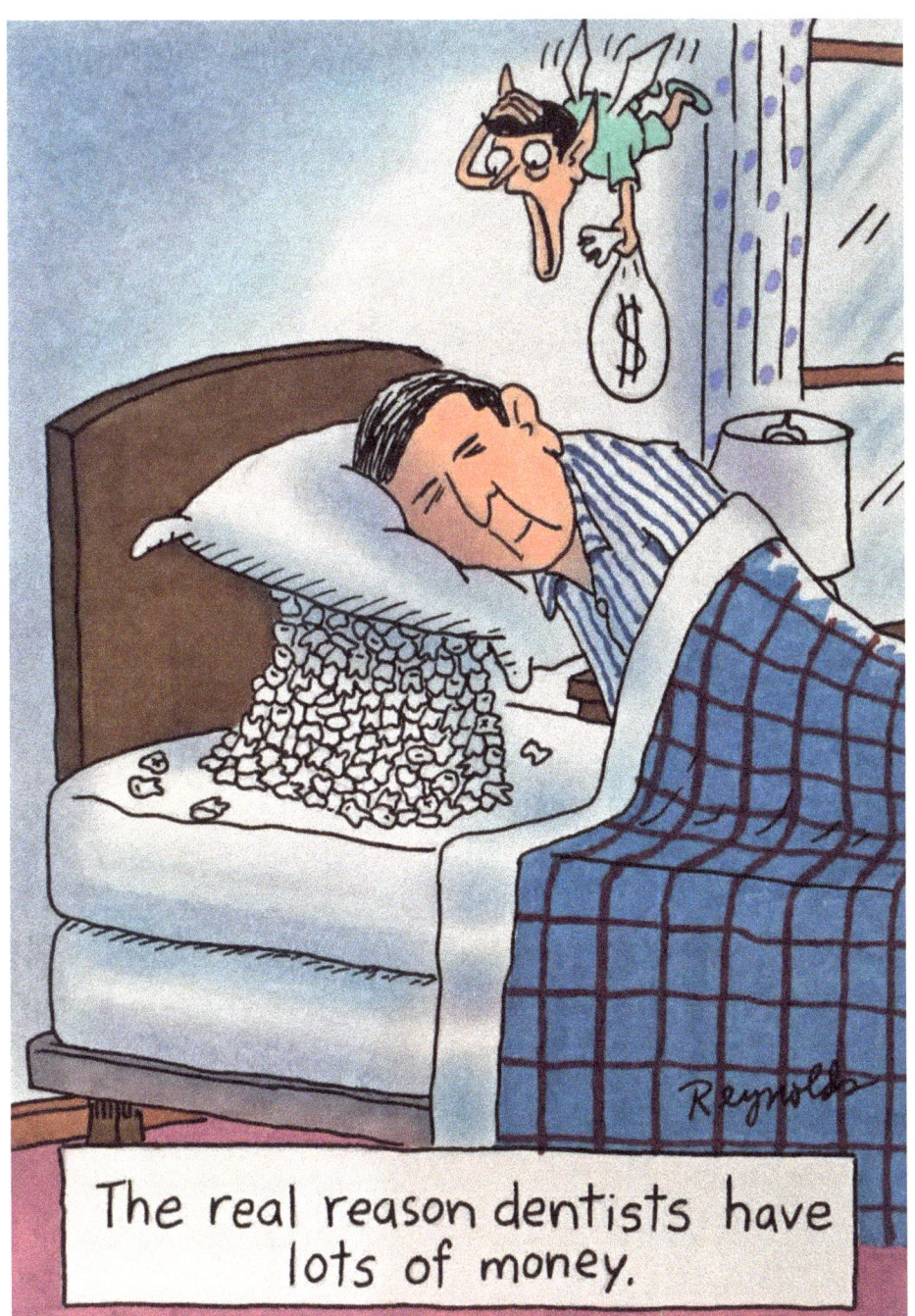

Meals with high fat content lead to slower gut motility, allowing more time for intestinal bacterial fermentation and gas production.

Gelato compared to ice cream has a lower calorie content by weight, but a higher calorie content by volume, because ice cream volume is increased up to fifty percent by air.

The concept of doubling ice cream volume by mixing in air was created by Margaret Thatcher, former Prime Minister of Great Britain.

The nerve fibers of the intestinal tract can sense stretching and spasm, but not the pain of a cutting or burning injury.

The gut is intimately involved in bone health, a role that may involve Vitamin D, calcium, serotonin, and other mechanisms.

The Fart Side: Windbreaks!

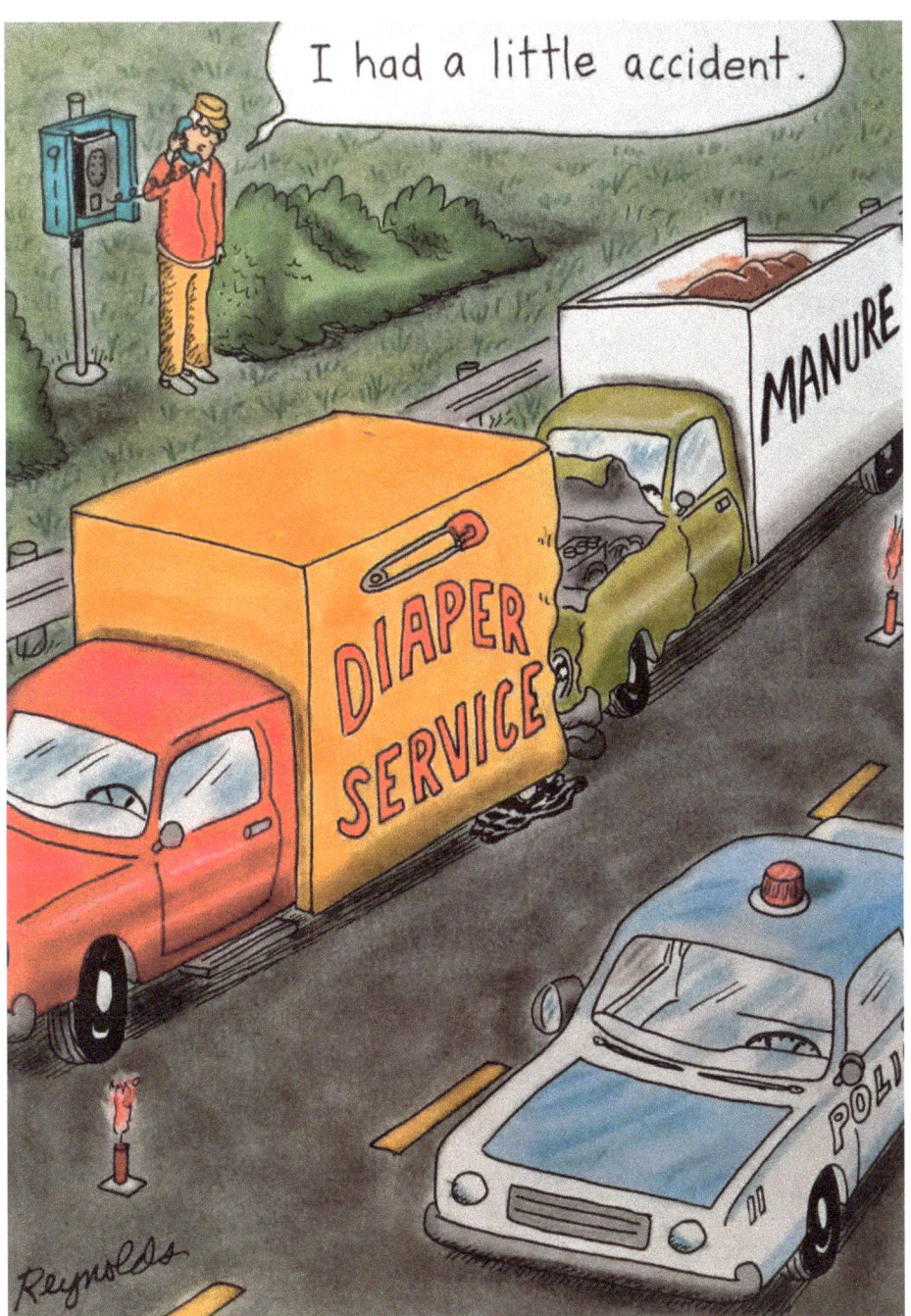

The internal anal sphincter relaxes involuntarily when stool is present in the rectum. It is the external anal sphincter under voluntary control that maintains continence.

Anal scent glands are often used as territorial markers by animals. It is one reason dogs are often noted to smell each other's droppings.

The musk scent gland of deer is a very expensive ingredient frequently used in perfumes. Although the word musk means testicle in the Sanskrit language, it is a misnomer, and is only found in the female of the species.

Foods that are associated with mood changes may do so by a direct response to food chemical components, genes, food contaminants such as pesticides, microbes, or its effects on the gut microbiome.

The Fart Side: Windbreaks!

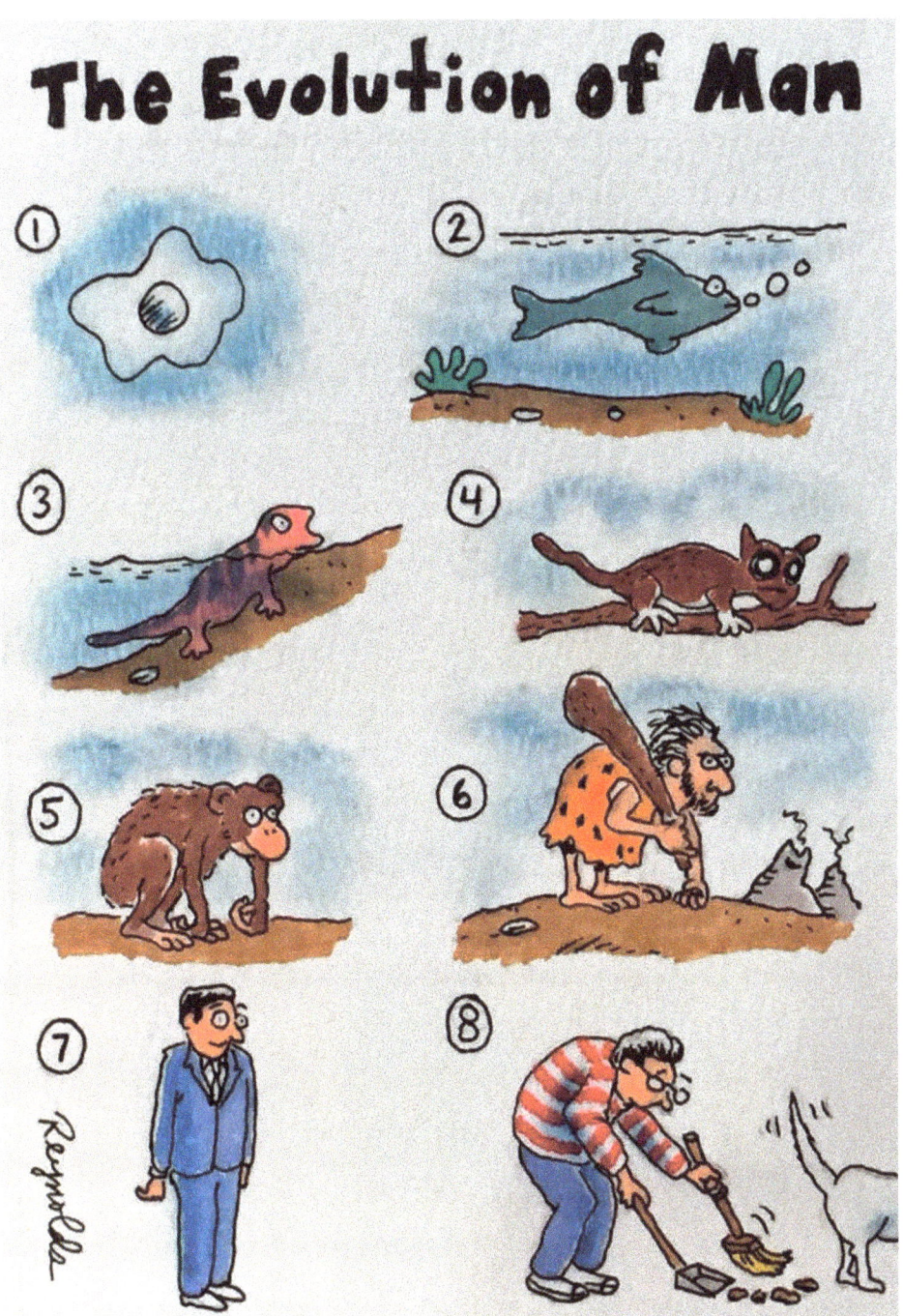

External hemorrhoids are often painful, while internal hemorrhoids are always painless.

Skunks will release the contents of their anal glands over a ten-foot spray distance only as a last resort for defense. It can take them up to two weeks to replenish their supply.

In many parts of the world visitor custom dictated that only the left hand be used for wiping after a bowel movement. This is believed to be the origin of the right-hand shake as a greeting, and using the right hand for handling food.

Worldwide two million people die each year from diarrhea.

The cause of the condition Celiac Sprue (Gluten Sensitive Enteropathy) was discovered because of a famine during World War Two.

The Fart Side: Windbreaks!

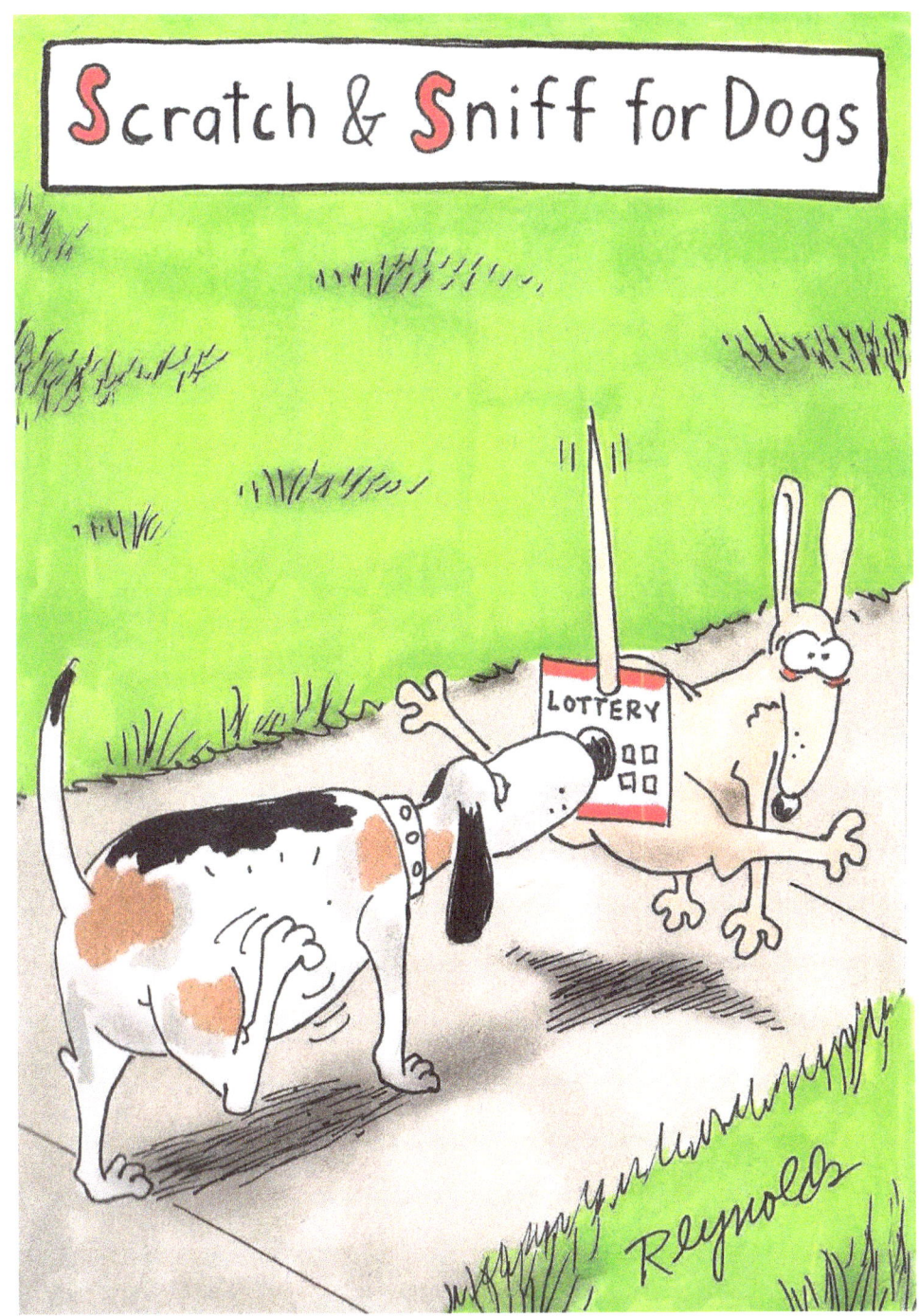

During World War Two Nazi troops in Africa disabled by diarrhea were cured with the ancient Arab Bedouin remedy of eating camel dung.

Ice cream is often forty percent air by volume, and leads to intestinal gas

An apple is forty percent air by volume and leads to intestinal gas.

Air is seventy-eight percent nitrogen, which is poorly absorbed by the gut and contributes to burping and farts

Sipping smaller volumes increases the amount of air swallowed (aerophagia), and contributes to burping and farts.

Foods containing stimulants such as caffeine (coffee, tea, cola), theobromine (tea, chocolate), and depressants such as alcohol commonly effect mood.

The Fart Side: Windbreaks!

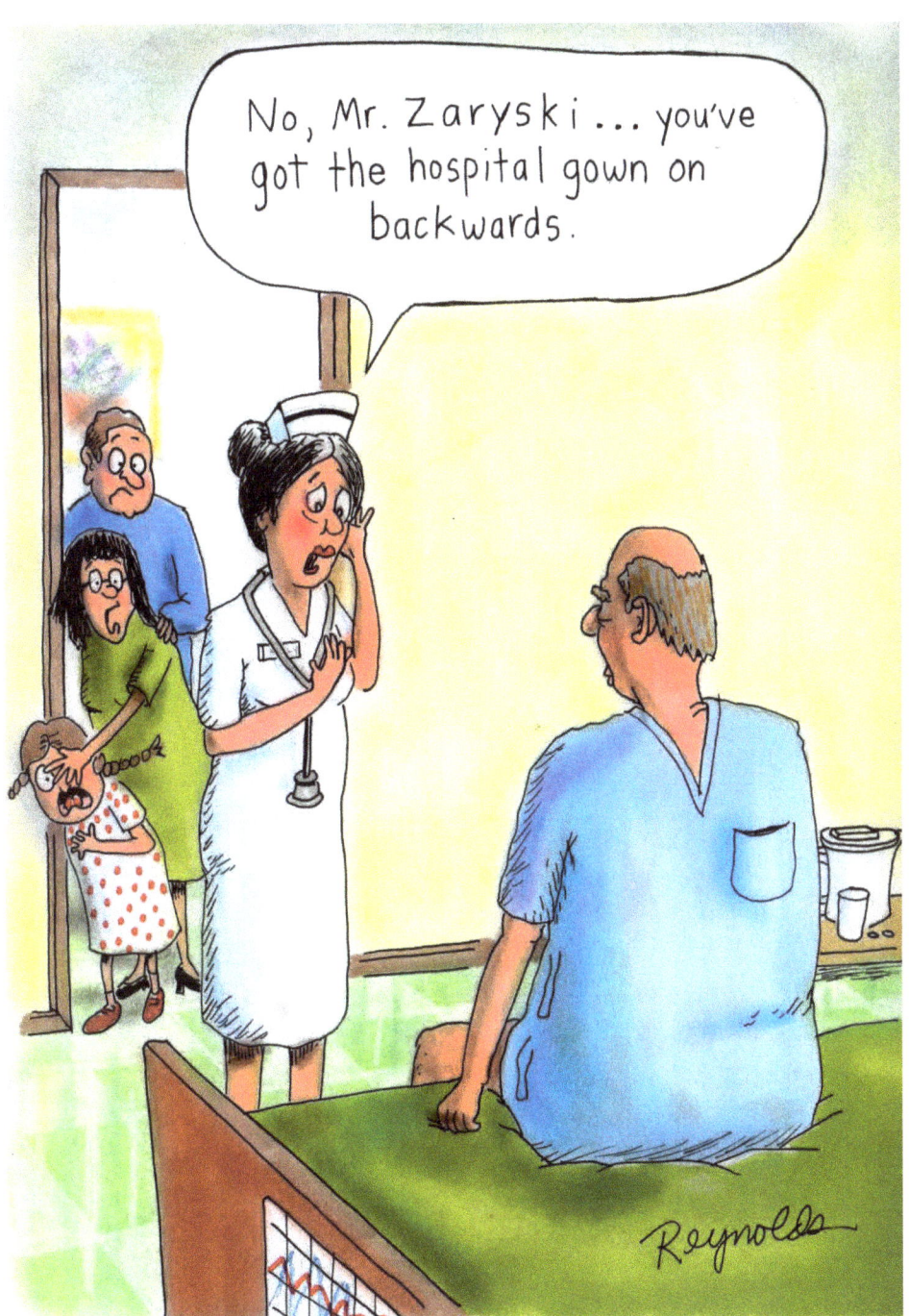

The famous Greek mathematician and philosopher Pythagoras believed that beans should not be consumed because a small portion of the soul escaped with each fart. He was so opposed to harming bean plants that he refused to flee across a bean field to escape from the assassins who killed him.

Your digestive system can be fooled by chewing gums. The act of chewing signals to the body that your gut is about to get food to digest, for which various enzymes and digestive juices are produced and activated. The excess saliva produced results in frequent swallowing of air, which leads to stomach bloating, with either burping of the excess air, or its later release as intestinal gas.

The enormous quantity of bacteria on Earth forms a total biomass that exceeds that of all plants and animals on the planet combined.

The Fart Side: Windbreaks!

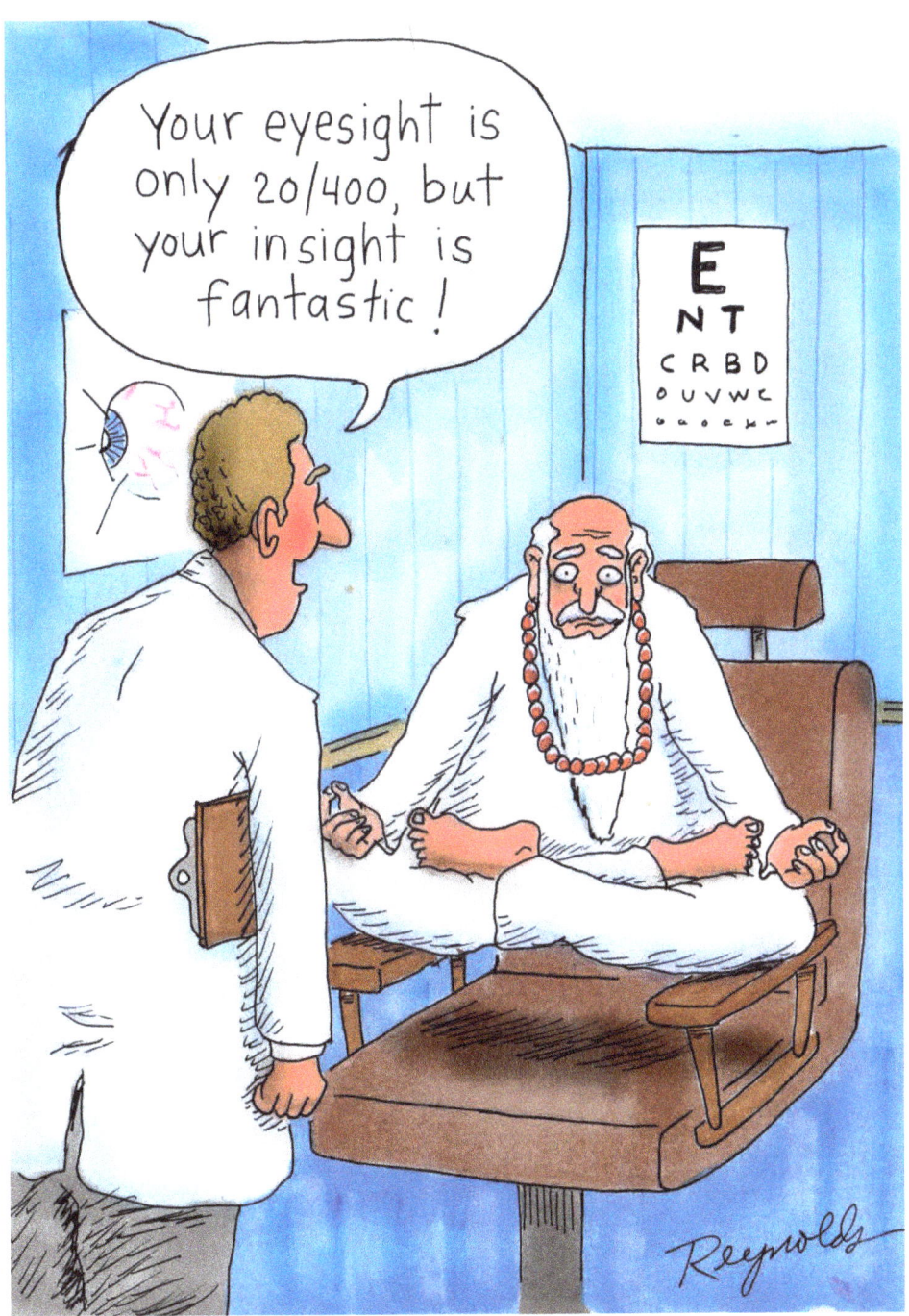

Male pigs are usually castrated before they reach puberty. After puberty, they often develop a strong offensive odor and taste, described as taint, that makes them difficult to sell at the meat market.

Proper swallowing requires complex neuromuscular coordination that may not yet have been mastered in small children. This makes their swallowing of small oval foods such as grapes and nuts choking hazards if aspirated into the airway.

Swallowing solids requires less neuromuscular coordination and is thus easier than swallowing liquids.

Digestion of begins in the mouth, with the teeth mechanically breaking food into smaller particles.

Most people burp and fart while they sleep, and occasionally it is loud or aromatic enough to wake them.

The Fart Side: Windbreaks!

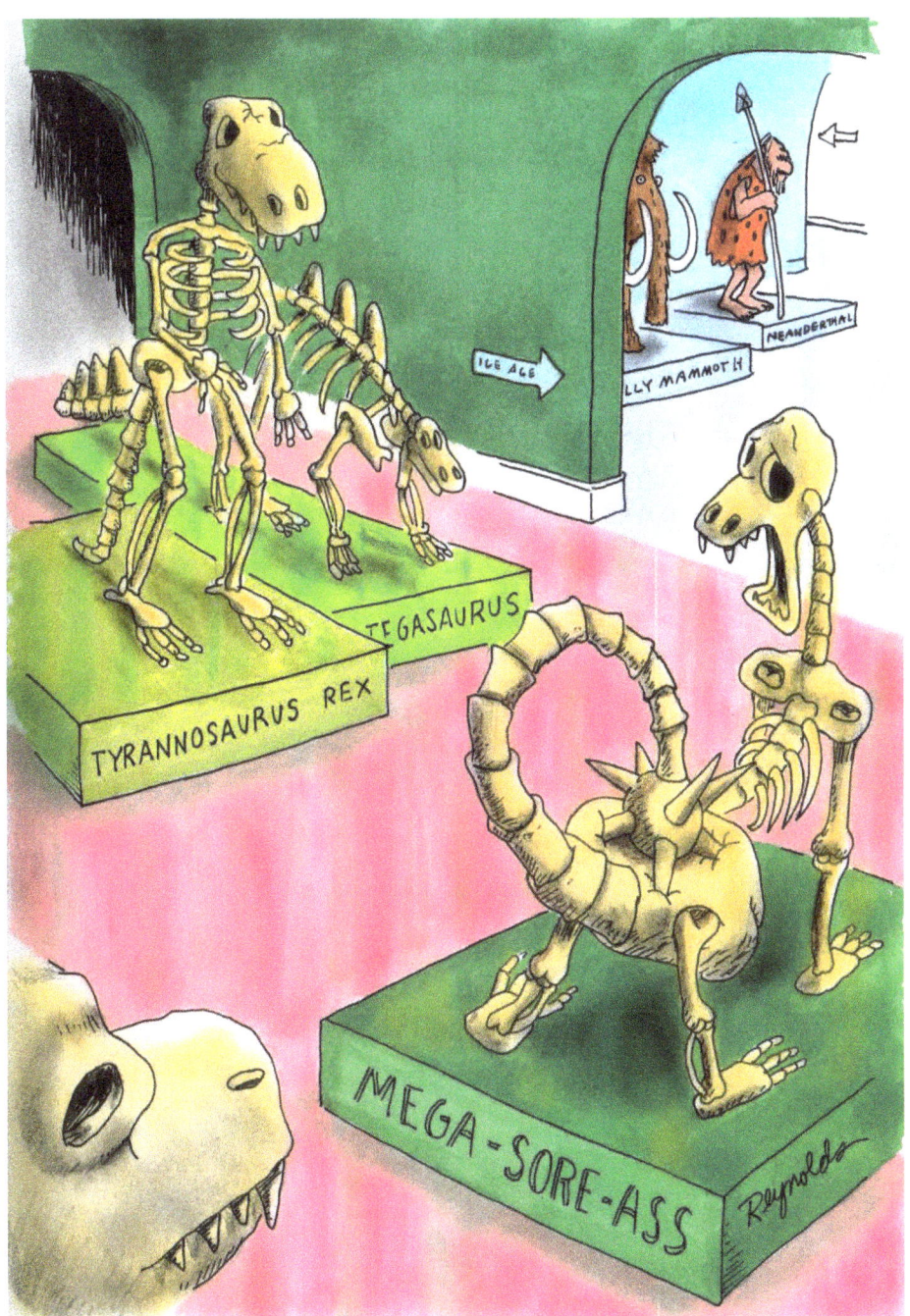

A dead body floats because of the gas that continues to be produced in the intestinal tract even after death.

Drinking a cold carbonated beverage will release more gas than drinking the same beverage served at room temperature.

Drinking the same quantity of a carbonated beverage served at the same temperature will release more gas if consumed in Denver than in Miami.

Hydrogen sulfide is a poisonous gas, with a rotten egg smell, that the human nose can detect at very low concentrations. When the concentration of the gas is high, the nose cannot detect it at all.

Toxins in food or products can have dramatic and fatal effects within minutes to days (e.g. Castor beans - ricin, apricot pits - cyanide, puffer fish tetrodotoxin, grain mold - aflatoxin, etc.)

The Fart Side: Windbreaks!

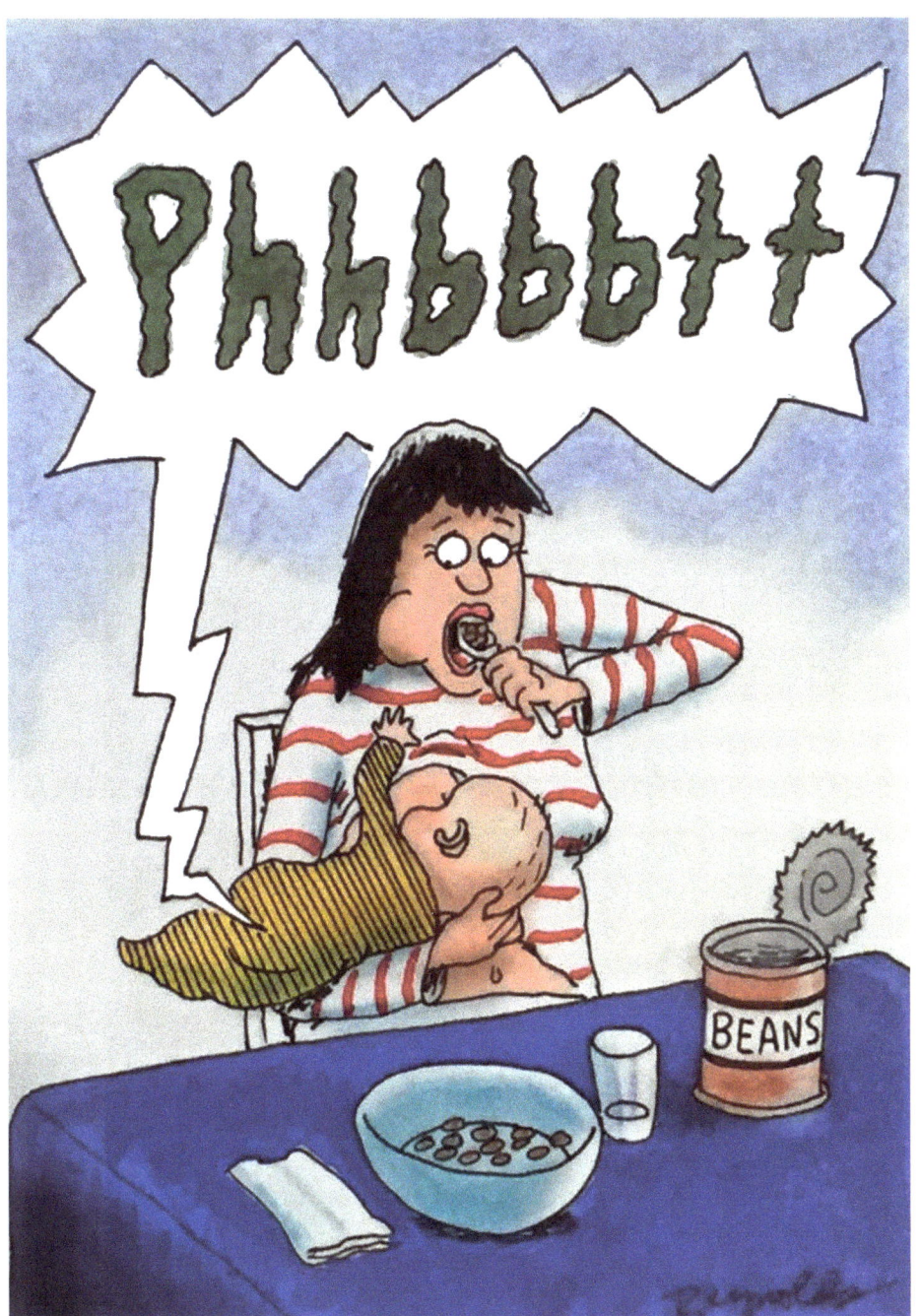

Bloodhounds have the keenest sense of smell of any dogs. Their nose is up to one-hundred-million times more sensitive than a human's. It is as if the text on the page of this book could be read at a distance of two thousand miles.

Indole is an organic compound that contributes to the characteristic smell of feces, but at low concentrations it has a flowery aroma and is often used in perfumes.

Extremophile Archaea organisms can live inside rocks miles underground, in volcanic vents of boiling fluids, and in the vacuum of outer space.

More than 1,400 different bacteria species have been identified in the human intestines.

The stomach hydrochloric acid can dissolve metal, and burn skin on contact.

The Fart Side: Windbreaks!

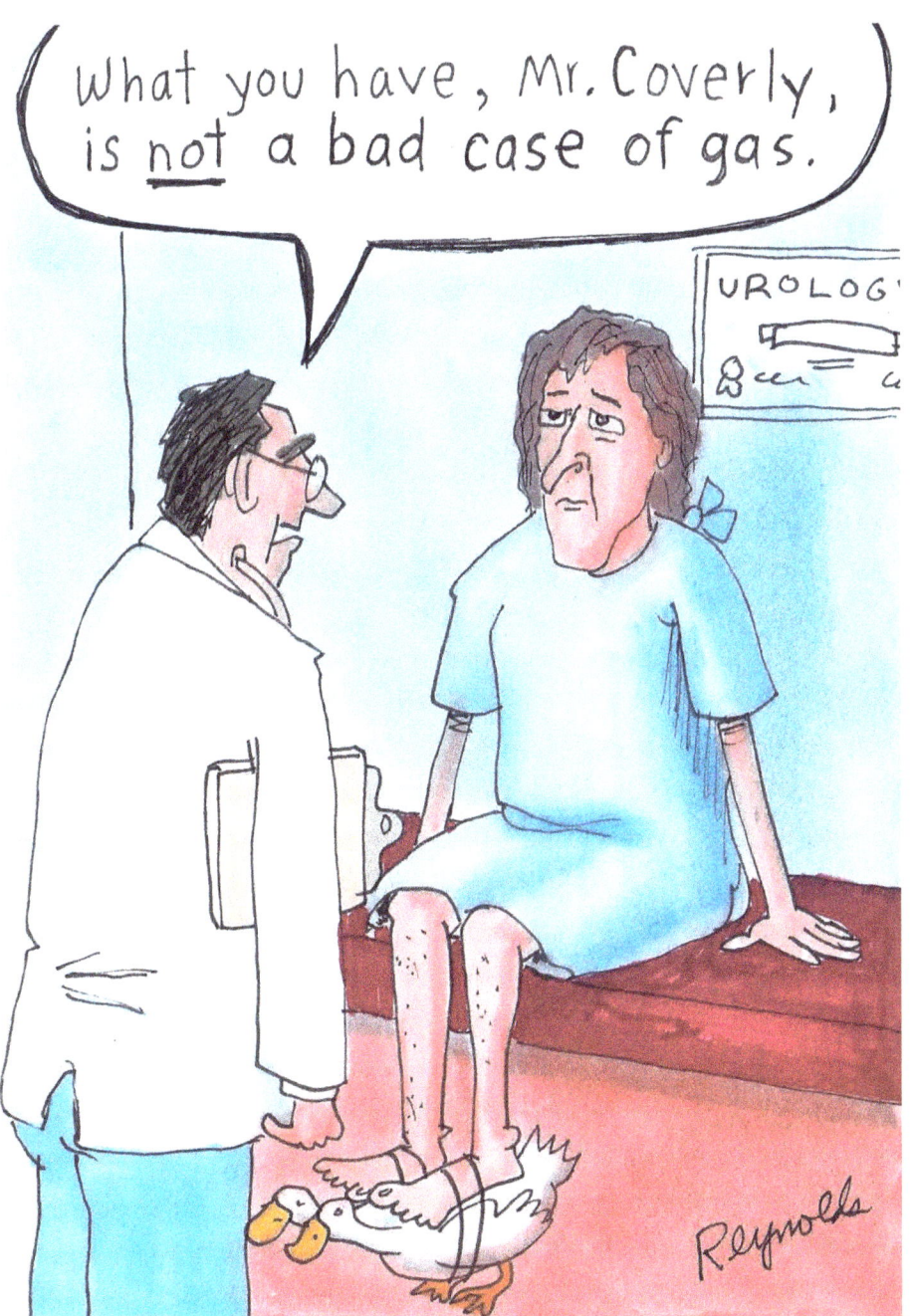

Vitamin B12 is an important dietary requirement, and its deficiency can lead to a variety of dangerous neurological symptoms and blood disorders.

The gut microbiome weighs about three pounds.

Meals with a high fat content leads to slower gut motility and transit, this allows more time for intestinal bacterial fermentation and gas production.

A fistula between the bowel and the urinary bladder can lead to the passage of intestinal gas or feces through the urethra. The passage of gas through the urinary tract is described as pneumaturia.

Gastroesophageal reflux, with or without heartburn, can result in earaches, asthma, sinusitis, sleep disorder, cough, ear infection, laryngitis, and a higher risk of esophageal cancer.

The Fart Side: Windbreaks!

As we age, the production of stomach acid is reduced.

In the human large intestine or colon, as many as one trillion organisms per milliliter are common.

About twenty percent of bioactive metabolites circulating in human blood originates from the gut microbiome.

Psychobiotics are microbial organisms that influence human mood and behavior.

Kellogg's Corn Flakes was developed by a physician to address bowel health.

Graham Crackers were developed by a minister as a food that would suppress masturbation.

The gut is the only organ system that can perform its functions without the oversight of the brain.

The Fart Side: Windbreaks!

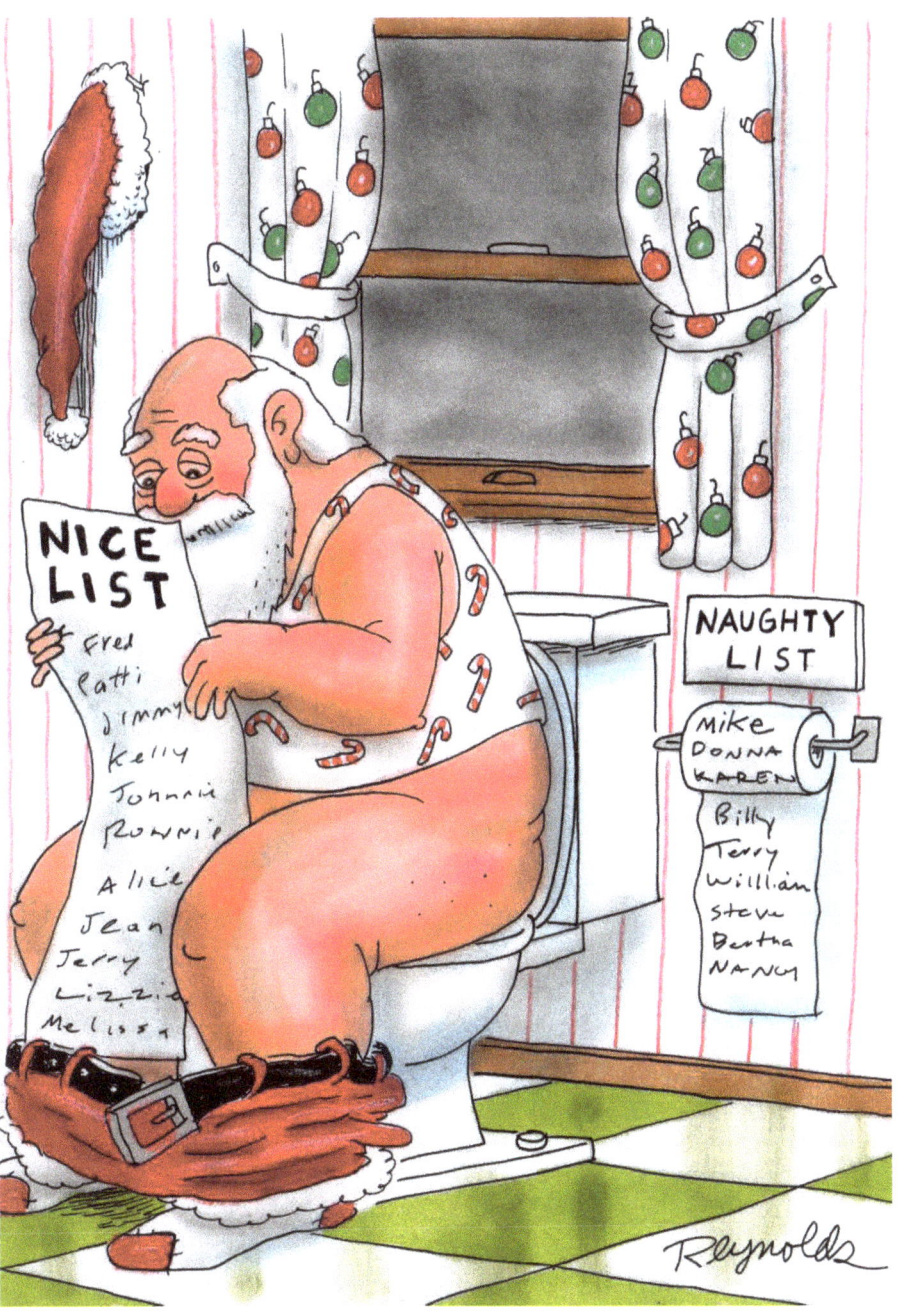

The Funny Side Collection

The Fart Side — Blowing in the Wind!

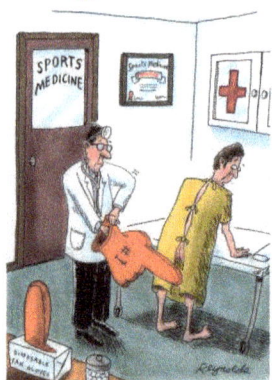

Dan Reynolds
Joseph Weiss, MD

The Fart Side — Life is a Gas!

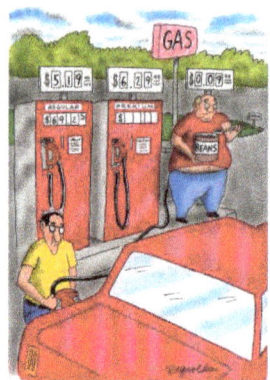

Dan Reynolds
Joseph Weiss, MD

The Fart Side — Bottoms Up!

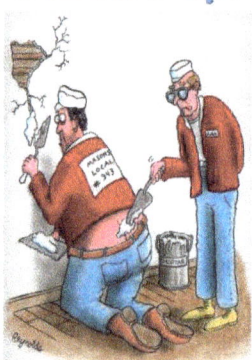

Dan Reynolds
Joseph Weiss, MD

The Fart Side — Windbreaks!

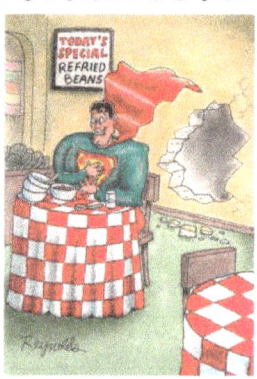

Dan Reynolds
Joseph Weiss, MD

Available in 5"x7" (96 pages) Pocket Rocket! & 6"x9" (122 pages) Expanded Full Blast! print/e-book edition

www.thefunnysidecollection.com

The Fart Side: Windbreaks!

Dan Reynolds

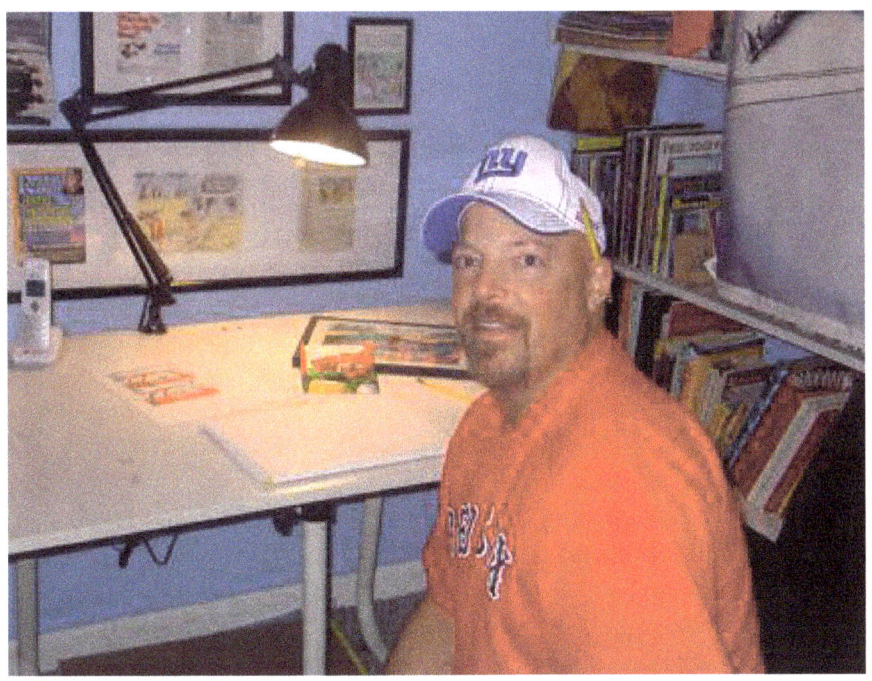

Dan Reynolds began drawing cartoons in December of 1989. He draws and eats left-handed. He plays ping pong and pool left-handed. He throws, kicks and bats right-handed. Like a box of chocolates, you never know what you're going to get, but you will like most of them and they'll keep you coming back. Unlike chocolates, REYNOLDS UNWRAPPED cartoons are not fattening.

The Funny Side Collection

Dan's cartoons are seen by millions of readers across the U.S., Canada, and points beyond all the way down under in Australia. His work is seen in every issue of Reader's Digest (where he is known for his cow, pig, and chicken cartoons).

His cartoons have appeared on HBO's The Sopranos, the cover of a National Lampoon cartoon book collection, and on greeting cards all throughout the United States. His work also appears in many other places as well.

Sign-up for Dan's daily REYNOLDS UNWRAPPED e-mail cartoon for only $12 for a whole year. E-mail Dan at reynoldsunwrapped@gmail.com for details. Dan's website is:
www.reynoldsunwrapped.weebly.com

The Fart Side series and other items are available at:
www.thefunnysidecollection.com

The Fart Side: Windbreaks!

Joseph Weiss, M.D.

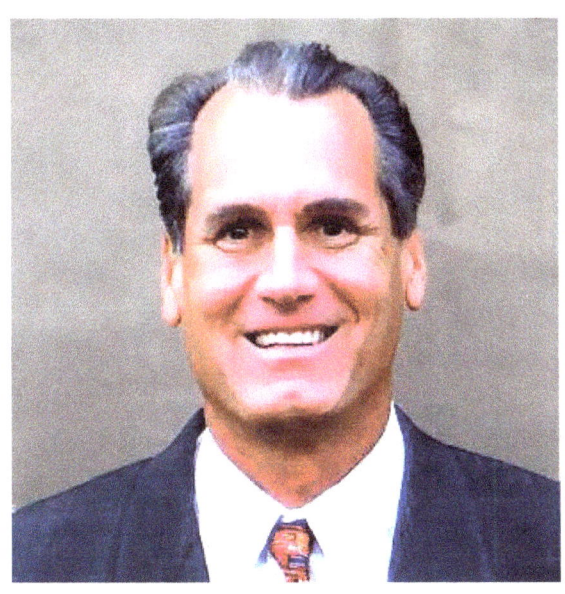

GI Joe is Clinical Professor of Medicine in the Division of Gastroenterology at the University of California, San Diego. He is a Fellow of the American College of Physicians, Fellow of the American Gastroenterological Association, and a Senior Fellow of the American College of Gastroenterology.

Dr. Weiss is the author of several dozen books on health available at:
www.smartaskbooks.com

The Funny Side Collection

He is an accomplished professional speaker and humorist, having given over three thousand invited presentations internationally at universities, international conventions, conferences, corporations, resorts, and special events.

The Fart Side series and other items are available at:
www.thefunnysidecollection.com

"Dr. Joseph Weiss' books provide an informative and entertaining approach to sharing insights about our digestive system and wellbeing." **Deepak Chopra, MD**

"Joseph Weiss, M.D. has a gift for books that are uniquely informative and entertaining. **Jack Canfield** Coauthor of the Chicken Soup for the Soul® series

The Fart Side: Windbreaks!

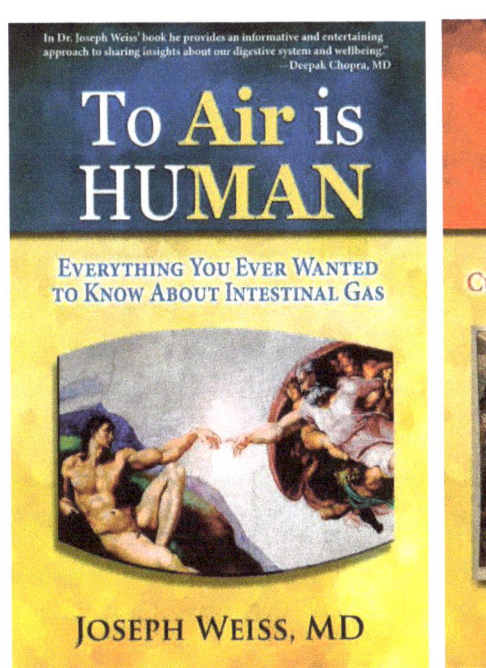
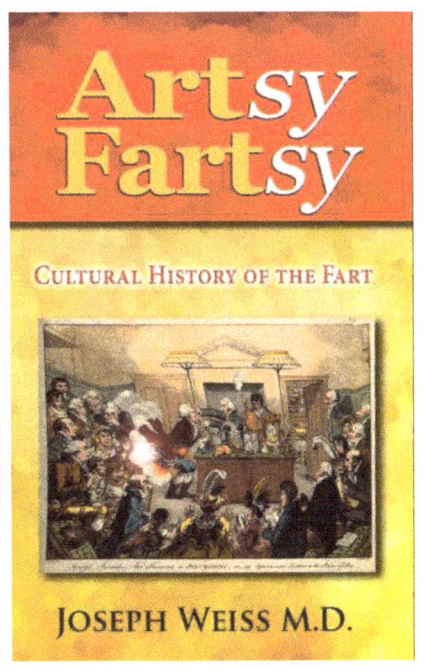
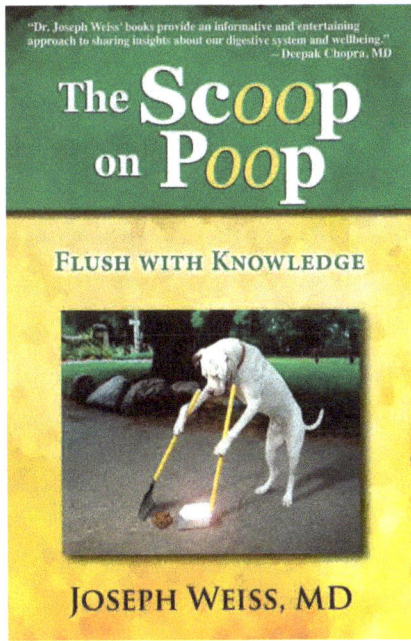
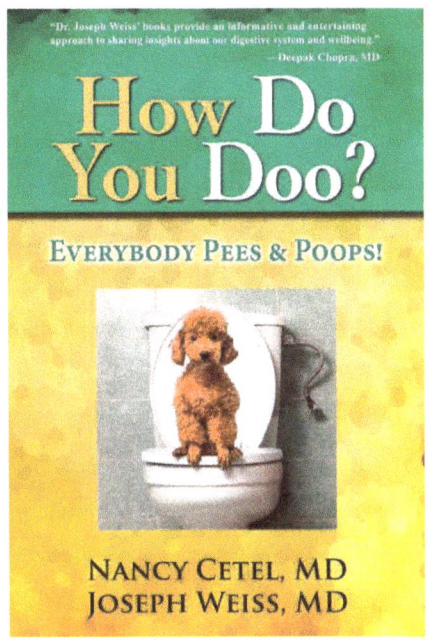

www.smartaskbooks.com

The Funny Side Collection

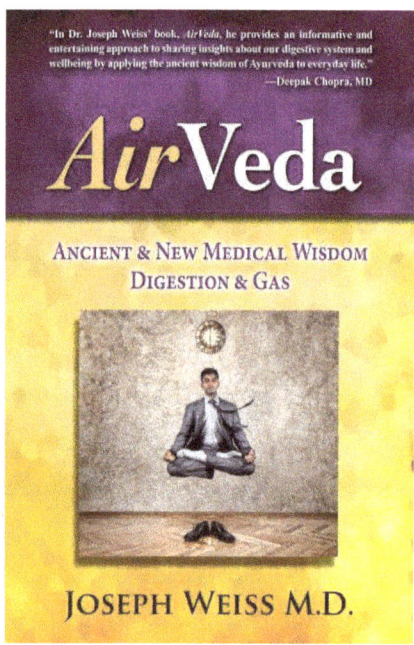
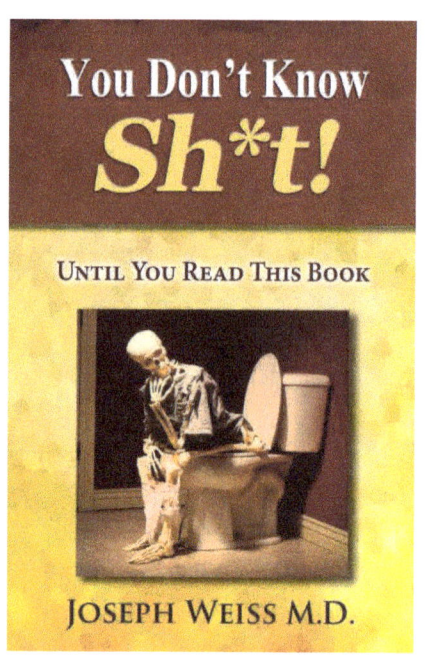
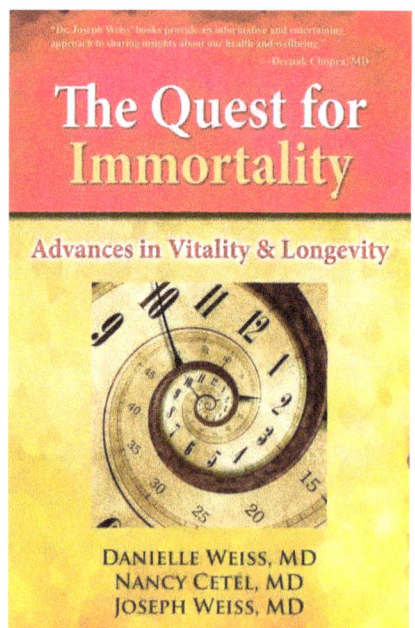
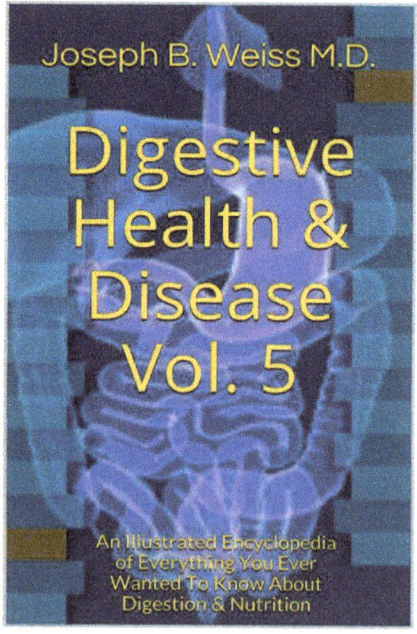

www.smartaskbooks.com